# Doctors in Fiction

# Doctors in Fiction
## Lessons from Literature

**BORYS SURAWICZ** M.D., M.A.C.C.
*Professor Emeritus of Medicine*
*University of Indiana School of Medicine*
*Past President, Association of University Cardiologists*
*Past President, American College of Cardiology*

and

**BEVERLY JACOBSON**
*Freelance Writer*

Radcliffe Publishing
Oxford • New York

**Radcliffe Publishing Ltd**
18 Marcham Road
Abingdon
Oxon OX14 1AA
United Kingdom

www.radcliffe-oxford.com
Electronic catalogue and worldwide online ordering facility.

British Library Cataloguing in Publication Data

A catalogue record for this book is available from the British Library.

ISBN-13: 978 184619 328 6

The paper used for the text pages of this book is FSC certified. FSC (The Forest Stewardship Council) is an international network to promote responsible management of the world's forests.

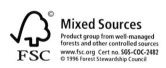

**Mixed Sources**
Product group from well-managed forests and other controlled sources
www.fsc.org Cert no. SGS-COC-2482
© 1996 Forest Stewardship Council

Typeset by Pindar NZ, Auckland, New Zealand
Printed and bound by TJI Digital, Padstow, Cornwall, UK

# Contents

# Preface

This book, assembled from notes on various works of fiction read by us over decades, is aimed principally at physicians, medical students and other members of the medical profession. Personal experience suggests that the professional life of a physician, particularly one with a family, does not leave much time to read fiction, except perhaps on vacation, when the most likely book taken along is a current best-seller or a popular mystery. The so-called classics are seldom picked up after the college years.

To this population of doctors and other medical personnel we are offering a collection of books with a unifying theme that should be of particular interest to them, namely how the medical profession is viewed by prominent writers and how their writings may affect the judgment of the medical profession by readers. We have tapped doctors from various periods of history, which offers some insight into the growing usefulness of medical practice, and observed that the phenomenal advances in medical science resulting in cures of numerous diseases, low infant mortality, effective public health measures and a markedly increased human life span in the developed countries have had no discernible effect on the relationship between doctor and patient.

Doctors are obliged to take the ancient or the modernized Hippocratic oath, which does not say anything about such ethical issues as excessive honoraria; fee splitting; superfluous medications; unnecessary procedures; accepting presents, dinners, travel and other expenses from drug companies; and large fees for expert testimonies in court cases. All of the above and other ethical transgressions are spotted by the writers and mercilessly exposed to readers with ensuing damage to the image of the profession. Other items highlighted by our selected writers include the hard road women experienced entering the medical profession, the heroism of doctors in the midst of epidemics, the varying approaches to psychiatric and psychosomatic conditions, the licensing of refugee physicians and the thorny issues of abortion and end-of-life care.

We fully realize that it would be improper to claim that the subject of doctors in literature is original to us. The similarly entitled monograph by Dr. Solomon Posen lists five books published between 1958 and 1993 on the subject of literature and medicine, and even more books and articles dealing with this topic can be found on the Internet. Dr. Posen's book contains quotations from about 600 works of literature featuring physicians selected by the author out of more than 1000 books with a "doctor as a principal figure."[1]

Although not in possession of such omnivorous knowledge of pertinent literature, we also had to perform arbitrary selections from the list of books read over time. It was easy to leave out fictional doctors such as Frankenstein, Jekyll, Faustus and the genial Dr. Watson of Dr. Conan Doyle, but considerable deliberation preceded the exclusion of doctors in such classics as Flaubert's *Madame Bovary*, Thomas Mann's *Magic Mountain*, Somerset Maugham's *Of Human Bondage*, Dostoyevsky's *Brothers Karamazov*, Joseph Conrad's *Nostromo* or Émile Zola's *Dr. Pascal* – for the reason that the doctor did not play a prominent role in the plot or that the practice of medicine was not the doctor's main interest in life. We also have dispensed with books deemed by us to be of lesser literary merit and thus less pleasurable to read. The offered menu consists, with few exceptions, of books by celebrated writers, seven of whom won the Nobel Prize in Literature.

We trust that our synopses and comments will entice the reader to make a closer acquaintance with their fictional colleagues immortalized in the literary works of prominent writers and at the same time provide pleasure from following interesting plots and enjoying tasteful prose.

**Borys Surawicz**
**Beverly Jacobson**
*January 2009*

## REFERENCE

1 Posen S. *The Doctor in Literature*. Oxford: Radcliffe Publishing; 2005. p. 3.

# About the authors

**Borys Surawicz** M.D., F.A.C.P., F.A.H.A., M.A.C.C. is a graduate of Stefan Batory University College of Medicine in Poland. He became a U.S. citizen in 1956. He is professor emeritus of medicine at the University of Kentucky College of Medicine, where he was director of the Cardiovascular Division of Medicine for 19 years, followed by a professorship at the Indiana University School of Medicine, where he was a senior associate at the Krannert Institute of Cardiovascular Research. He ended his professional career as an attending physician at the St. Vincent Hospital in Indianapolis, Indiana. He is past president of the Association of University Cardiologists and past president of the American College of Cardiology, an author of 280 peer-reviewed scientific papers, an editor of four and an author of two textbooks of cardiac electrophysiology and electrocardiography. He is listed as an educator in the current edition of Marquis *Who's Who in America*.

**Beverly Jacobson** received her B.A. from Mount Holyoke College, where she was elected to the Phi Beta Kappa Society. Her first career was as a wife and mother, raising five children. In 1973 she started freelancing, contributing articles on women's issues, women's health, parenting, joint custody, autism and the importance of discipline in raising children to *McCall's*, the *Ladies Home Journal*, *Redbook*, *Good Housekeeping*, *Parade*, *Parents*, *Woman's Day*, *Woman's World*, *Self* and the Westchester section of the *New York Times*. She is the author or co-author of six books, including *Women's Health Research*, written in collaboration with the Society for Women's Health Research; *Genetic Nutrition: Designing a Diet Based on Your Family Medical History*, with Victor Herbert M.D. and Artemis P. Simopoulos M.D.; and *Y2K and YOU: The Sane Person's Home-Preparation Guide*, with Dermot McGuigan.

## PART ONE

# Early docs

# CHAPTER 1

# Dr. Vesuvia Adelia Rachel Ortese Aguilar

## in *Mistress of the Art of Death*

by Ariana Franklin[1]

---

### Themes

- Salerno, a city that defies the perceived image of the Dark Ages by its embrace of religious tolerance, liberty, diverse culture and secular education
- Dr. Vesuvia Adelia Rachel Ortese Aguilar, an accomplished early female coroner
- The struggle of women for recognition and equality in the field of medicine
- The rise and fall of witchcraft trials

---

Here comes our earliest doctor – Vesuvia Adelia Rachel Ortese Aguilar – a 12th-century graduate of the Schola Medica Salernitana, the first known medieval medical school, located in the southern Italian town of Salerno in the Kingdom of Sicily. When we first encountered Adelia, as she is familiarly known in the novel, we thought the author was engaged in some apocryphal feminist joke. After all, in 12th-century Europe the proper place for a woman was in the home or the nunnery, and women who tried to cure people were sometimes accused of witchcraft. So how dare Franklin come up with an accomplished and sophisticated female medical doctor in 1171, when the opportunities for women to practice medicine did not exist in the Western world until the 19th century?

Of course we were wrong. Ariana Franklin is a medieval scholar, journalist and experienced researcher who, under her real name, Diana Norman, has written 13 respected historical novels, one of which, *Fitzempress' Law*, was cited by the BBC Radio Bookshelf as the best example of an historical novel for 1980. She is married to the film critic and broadcaster Barry Norman and lives with him and their two daughters in Hertfordshire.[2] *Mistress of the Art of Death* won the CWA Ellis Peters Historical Award in 2007.[3]

Salerno was a special place in the Middle Ages, where freedom of speech, religious practice and literacy were considered a Sicilian's birthright. It was a cosmopolitan city peopled by Muslims, Byzantines, Normans, Greeks and Jews. No wonder, then, that along with beautiful Romanesque architecture and true multiculturalism, an advanced medical school appeared. At this school, the works of notable early Greek physicians were taught, among them Hippocrates, known as the father of the medical profession and creator of the Hippocratic oath that set standards of medical ethics still guiding today's physicians; Galen, the great 1st-century physician and surgeon; and Dioscurides, whose *De Materia Medica* of the same time was an important compilation of the medical uses of plants. In fact the Salerno school, founded in a 9th-century monastery, hit its golden age between the 10th and 13th centuries, just in time to welcome the fictional Adelia.

But there are real life examples of early female doctors. Trotula di Ruggiero, born in 1090, was another physician at the Salerno Medical School and the author of *Passionibus Mulierum* (*The Diseases of Woman*).[4] Even earlier in antiquity women practiced midwifery and healing. For example, in 400 BC Greece, Hippocrates was instructing them in gynecology and obstetrics at his school in Asia Minor. Of course, all was not smooth sailing even in enlightened Greece. Athenian lawmakers learned that women were performing abortions and banned them from practicing medicine, imposing the death penalty for violators. Losing their female doctors and feeling uncomfortable taking their intimate health problems to male physicians, Greek women's mortality rate rose. In 300 BC a woman named Agnodice had to disguise herself as a man in order to study medicine at the great Alexandria University and continued wearing male garb after returning to Athens, where she set up a practice treating women. Her male colleagues, jealous of her success, charged her with corrupting women patients. When she revealed that she was a woman, she faced death. But the Athenian women saved her, going to the judges *en masse*, calling for her acquittal, which would allow her to continue practicing.[5] Although some believe Agnodice to be a mythical character, all this makes Adelia's novelistic career somewhat more believable.

## THE STORY

Adelia, an orphan raised by an atheist Jewish doctor, is a medical student but not an unusual one, as women students and teachers were regularly admitted to the Salerno Medical School. She has mastered the art of death, which today we call forensic medicine, making her, historically, the earliest fictional female coroner likely to turn up in any novel. She is calmly looking forward to a life of teaching, research and solving crimes in her home city when history intervenes. A series of terrible child murders in the English town of Cambridge has been blamed on the local Jews, who seek protection from King Henry II and are hiding in Cambridge Castle. Loath to sacrifice the income from taxes paid by prosperous Jewish merchants, Henry wishes to shield them from harm and appeals to his fellow royal and cousin, the King of Sicily, to send his best master of this frightful new science to help find the real killer(s), which should exonerate the Jews. But in backward England a woman doctor is unheard of and any female openly engaging in curative measures might be labeled a witch. Therefore, Adelia must travel with two companions, Mansur, a Muslim, who is really her bodyguard, and Simon of Naples, a clever and quick-witted Jew chosen to establish the innocence of his English co-religionists. Their combined detective work forms the essence of the story.

### Adelia's medical knowledge

As the three Sicilians travel towards Cambridge with a group of English pilgrims, Adelia's medical competence is quickly tested. Prior Geoffrey of St. Augustine's canonry of Barnwell is suffering great pain from urinary retention and is unable to walk. When his attendants, asking to borrow the cart in which the odd-looking threesome are traveling, discover inadvertently that one of them is a doctor and assume, of course, that it is Simon, they bring the overweight and suffering prior to him for help. Hiding the cart in the woods so that no one can view the procedure, Adelia, guarded by Mansur and helped by Simon, uses a sturdy reed plucked from a nearby stream as a medieval catheter to successfully relieve the blockage in the prior's urethra, even though she has never before done the procedure, having only heard of it from her stepfather. Her knowledge of male anatomy is clear when she warns her partially recovered patient the next day that the retention could happen again.

> "Men have a gland that is accessory to the male generative organs. It surrounds the neck of the bladder and the commencement of the urethra. In your case I believe it to be enlarged. Yesterday it pressed so hard that the bladder could not function."[6]

She offers to show him how to use the reed if needed, which he eschews, and advises him to eat less and exercise. (It seems this staple of medical advice has been given out by physicians for centuries.) The benefit of this encounter, however, is clear; Adelia and company have acquired a powerful protector in Prior Geoffrey.

Once in Cambridge, the prior arranges for Adelia to examine the remains of the murdered children so that she can determine how they were killed. This she does secretly, although she is watched by Sir Rowley Picot, King Henry's tax collector and ex-Crusader, whom she quickly puts to work helping her.

Prior Geoffrey also arranges for the Sicilians to live in one of the cottages abandoned by the Jews. He even supplies a local servant, the wily woman Gylthia and her grandson, Ulf, who are valuable in explaining local customs and personalities. No sooner do they move in than the locals assume that Mansur, wearing a traditional kaffiyeh, is the doctor, Arab medicine being well regarded even here, and immediately start asking for help for their various ills. Thus a new medical practice is born and serves as an excellent cover while Adelia and Simon continue their investigation of the child murders.

Adelia remains involved in treating the locals, quietly imparting her knowledge to the fake doctor Mansur. The remedies and procedures she uses include an eyewash of weak, strained agrimony on the infected and inflamed eyes of an old, nearly blind woman; amputating the gangrenous foot of a young man, using a cloth soaked in opium as an anesthetic, then stitching the edge of the wound and bandaging it. Meanwhile Dr. Mansur, now puffed up with his new importance, prescribes sugar for a child with a cough. Furious at this useless advice, Adelia substitutes an inhalation of essence of pine, which she maintains should help the youngster if his lungs are not too badly damaged.

Not all of her efforts are successful, because these patients come to the "foreign doctor" too late, so that the child with the cough develops pneumonia and a man with the ague dies, as does a new mother who hemorrhaged after delivery.

Perhaps Adelia's greatest medical accomplishment is saving Sir Rowley Picot from death after a brawl, during which a cleaver in his groin struck an artery, causing a major bleed. Putting her fist in the wound to plug off the site of hemorrhage then closing the wound on the proverbial kitchen table with thread and needle from the sheriff's wife's sewing kit may stretch the reader's credulity somewhat, particularly as Adelia is not sure during the procedure if she extracted all the pieces of his tunic from the wound, which would inevitably have caused infection and death from gangrene. Why was Sir Rowley brawling? We cannot reveal the cause except to say he was behaving heroically and that we must bear with the author, as Sir Rowley needs to survive to play a pivotal role in the denouement of this story and in solving its central crime. To say more would ruin the ending for the reader.

Meanwhile Adelia's doctoring is not over. A sickness has attacked the Saint Radegund's nunnery, where no man may enter. Adelia must go, pretend to report to Dr. Mansur and do his bidding. Plague is the rumor but Adelia thinks it is cholera, and a less virulent form than found in the east. She is faced with 20 vomiting, diarrheal nuns, a verminous kitchen and a resentful prioress who could not care less. Nevertheless, by using opium to ease the nuns' pain and calf's-foot jelly to nourish her patients, all but two of the nuns survive.

Finally, Ulf, who has become dear to her, disappears and Adelia goes to find him. In the course of this search the reader learns the identity of the monster child-killer and witnesses his flamboyant, over-the-top finish. But that is not the end of the novel, which twists and turns in very satisfactory ways. Remarkable Adelia is rewarded, we won't say how, the conflict between church and state is illuminated, and King Henry II, known throughout history primarily as the murderer of Thomas à Becket, comes off very well as a sly and crafty but decent king, whose gift to his country of trial by jury started England on the road to fairness and justice.

## SALERNO IN THE MIDDLE AGES

It should be obvious that we have selected this medieval murder mystery not for its literary prominence but primarily for the presence of a capable woman physician in 12th-century Europe. The acquired medical theoretical knowledge and practical skill of this woman is not a coincidence. Her acceptance as a physician required a cultural milieu that was unusual for her time. It is described by an historian, whose name happens to be Vincenzo Salerno, in his article in *Best of Sicily* magazine. He claimed that throughout the Norman era (roughly from AD 1070 to 1200) Sicilian society was more sophisticated than that which the Normans encountered in England or even mainland Italy. The polyglot culture of the Arabs and Byzantines was a prosperous intellectual, artistic and economic environment at the center of the most important region of the Mediterranean. It was a geographic crossroads between north and south, east and west. More important than this was the evolution of the social fabric of Norman Sicily, adapting essentially Arab institutions to European realities. The ethnic and religious tolerance was generally accepted as an integral part of Sicilian society, and multicultural co-existence usually prevailed. Nowadays, nations such as Canada, the United States and Australia seem to represent the epitome of tolerant, multicultural societies. In the Middle Ages, however, the concept was a novel one.[7]

This broad-minded, open society accepted women as equal to men, fostering their talents and aspirations. But the subsequent lessons from European history in the 600 years that followed the Salerno phenomenon teach us that a climate of religious intolerance, bigotry and cultural poverty coincides with the denigration of women and their exclusion from intellectual pursuits. We see this again in our own time in nations where extremist Islamic factions, such as the Taliban in Afghanistan, prohibit women from working or attending schools other than for religious study after the age of eight; remove women's voices from radio, television or public gatherings; ban them from leaving their houses unless accompanied by a male relative; and require them to wear garb that covers the entire body from head to foot.

## DARK AGES AND WITCHCRAFT

Barbara Ehrenreich and Deirdre English document the history of women's exclusion from medicine during the period between the 13th and 19th centuries.[8] Noting that women have always been healers – as midwives, abortionists, nurses, counselors and pharmacists, thanks to their knowledge of healing herbs – they call them "doctors without degrees." The exclusion of women was part of a deliberate male takeover of the medical profession and, the authors maintain, the first stage of this attack was the burning of witches, women who were lay healers serving the poor.

In earlier centuries the medieval Church was not interested in witches, largely because it had accepted the view of St. Augustine, who, in the early 400s AD, argued that God alone could suspend the normal laws of the universe. Two events started the Church on a new road: Pope Innocent III's attack on the Cathar sect as heretic in 1208 because its members accepted supernatural powers, and Thomas Aquinas' belief in "dangerous demons." These developments led directly to the witchcraft trials which erupted in the 14th and 15th centuries. In fact, Pope Innocent VIII commissioned two friars, Heinrich Kramer and Jacob Sprenger, to investigate suspected witchcraft, and the result, the *Malleus Maleficarum* (*Hammer of Witches*), published in 1484, replaced St. Augustine's benign view of the supernatural with a new orthodoxy which taught that Christians had to hunt down and kill witches. The fact that this book was reprinted 13 times in the next 40 years lends weight to its importance in keeping alive the witchcraft trials that flourished between 1374 and 1682, when the last witch was executed in England. This doctrine then jumped the Atlantic to Salem, Massachusetts, where, in a climate of absolute hysteria, 19 witches were hung in 1692.[9]

It is clear that the society of the Middle Ages came to believe in the reality of witches as much as modern society believes in the reality of atoms, even though we can't see them. However, we cannot find any evidence that the witch-hunts that occurred between the 14th and 17th centuries in Europe were directed specifically against female lay healers, although it is estimated that 80% of those killed were women. Also, Ehrenreich and English's stated numbers of witch-hunt victims in the millions is wildly overblown. More sober estimates put the figure around 40,000 witches, a disturbing enough number in its own right.[10]

## FIRST WOMEN PHYSICIANS

It was not until the 19th century that women started returning to the medical field. In the United States the popular health movement of the 1830s and 40s led to Ladies Physiological Societies, which gave courses in anatomy and personal hygiene, advising frequent bathing, comfortable loose clothing and a wholesome diet.

The first woman doctor we've found in the United States was Elizabeth Blackwell (1821–1910). She received a medical degree from the Geneva Medical College in New York, practiced obstetrics and gynecology and co-founded the New York Infirmary for Women in 1857, which, along with the medical school begun in 1867, provided training opportunities for women doctors and medical care for the poor.[11] Another medical pioneer in the United States was Dr. Mary Edwards Walker (1832–1919), who was refused permission to work as a physician during the Civil War, even though she had earned a genuine medical degree from Syracuse Medical College in 1853 and wore men's clothing. She was relegated to nursing and spying but finally received a commission as an army surgeon in 1863, becoming the first female surgeon in the U.S. Army. She was awarded the Congressional Medal of Honor on November 11, 1865, which needed a special bill signed by then President Andrew Johnson. She is the only woman ever to receive this award. A postage stamp honoring her was issued in 1982.[12]

In England, Elizabeth Garrett Anderson (1836–1917) studied privately and only with great difficulty obtained a degree from the Society of Apothecaries, which entitled her to a place on the medical register. She was the first woman in Britain to achieve this status. In 1866 she became a general medical attendant at St. Mary's Dispensary, where poor women could consult doctors of their own gender, and later received an M.D. from the University of Paris in 1870. St. Mary's evolved into the New Hospital for Women, where Dr. Garrett worked for over 20 years.[13]

By the early 20th century only midwifery remained a female prerogative in the United States; in 1910 nearly 50% of all babies were delivered by midwives. These women were repeatedly attacked as incompetent by the medical profession, which blamed them for the high incidence of puerperal sepsis and ophthalmia, allowing men to take control of obstetrical care and move birth from the home to the hospital. In Europe, however, midwifery training was upgraded and appropriate techniques were taught, such as hand washing for prevention of puerperal sepsis and eye drops for ophthalmia, which allowed midwives to be recognized as members of an acceptable profession.

Today, when nearly half of all medical school students are female, it is important to remember the dark past and the struggles of early pioneers who slowly, with great difficulty and considerable bravery, started pushing open the heavy iron doors barring women from medical practice.

## REFERENCES

1 Franklin A. *Mistress of the Art of Death*. New York: GP Putnam and Sons; 2007.
2 Book Browse. *Ariana Franklin*. Available at: www.bookbrowse.com/biographies/index.cfm?author_number=1527
3 Edwards, M. *Ariana Franklin*. Available at: www.doyouwriteunderyourownname.blogspot.com/2008/05/ariana-franklin.html
4 Green MH, editor. *The Trotula: a medieval compilation of women's medicine*. Philadelphia: University of Pennsylvania Press; 2001.
5 Lienhard JH. *Early Women Doctors* in Engines of our Ingenuity Website: Available at: www.uh.edu/engines/. Copyright 1988–1997.
6 Franklin, op. cit., pp. 46–7.
7 Salerno V. Sicilian peoples: the Normans. *Best of Sicily*. 2005. Available at: www.bestofsicily.com/mag/art171.htm
8 Ehrenreich B, English D. *Witches, Midwives and Nurses: a history of women healers*. New York: The Feminist Press at the City University of New York; 1970.
9 Linder D. *A Brief History of Witchcraft Persecution Before Salem*. Available at: www.law.umkc.edu/faculty/projects/ftrials/salem/witchhistory.html
10 Hutton R. *The Triumph of the Moon: a history of modern pagan witchcraft*. New York: Oxford University Press; 2000.
11 National Library of Medicine. *Dr. Elizabeth Blackwell*. Available at: www.nlm.nih.gov/changingthefaceofmedicine/physicians/biography_35.html
12 *Woman of Courage Profile* written and produced by the St. Lawrence County N.Y. Branch of The American Association of University Women (AAUW).
13 www.spartacus.schoolnet.co.uk/WandersonE.htm

# CHAPTER 2

# Dr. Stephen Maturin

## in *The Aubrey-Maturin Chronicles*
### by Patrick O'Brian[1]

---

### Themes

- Seafaring naval surgeon Dr. Stephen Maturin is also a naturalist, linguist, musician and spy
- Naval medicine in Great Britain during the Napoleonic Wars

---

This long-running and popular naval saga, considered by some critics as comprising the best historical novels ever written, features the adventures of an oddly matched pair of characters at the beginning of the 19th century. The tall, stout, handsome Jack Aubrey, son of an admiral, is an officer in the Royal Navy. He is a daring, courageous and inspiring leader, a seaman since boyhood, beloved by his crew but not very savvy on land and without an inquisitive mind when it comes to business and politics.

Dr. Stephen Maturin is a short, slender, highly intellectual physician, but a landlubber with little interest in navigation, often stumbling and falling while stepping from the barge onto the deck of a ship. They meet in Port Mahon, where Lieutenant Aubrey, depressed, poor and without a ship, finally receives his first command: the relatively small 14-gun brig-rigged HM Sloop *Sophie*. Maturin is also in Mahon, hard on his luck and without a job. Their encounter takes place at a recital where Maturin offends Aubrey when he asks him to stop tapping his foot to the music, since he is half a beat off. But when they meet again Stephen accepts Jack's offer to be a surgeon on his new command. Thus begins a friendship that will last through the course of their adventures, vividly pictured in 20 book installments beginning with *Master and*

*Commander*, published in 1969, and ending with *Blue at the Mizzen*, published in 1999, shortly before O'Brian's death. (A 21st novel restored from a partial collection of chapters left by O'Brian has been published under the title *The Final Unfinished Voyage of Jack Aubrey*.) These stories span the period of the Napoleonic Wars from 1800 to 1817, with Aubrey commanding 17 different ships and rising in rank from lieutenant to admiral. The reader following the ships crisscrossing the oceans, with frequent landings on the different shores of the five continents, is rewarded with a geographical survey of our planet 200 years ago, when it was still largely in pristine condition and not despoiled by fossil-fuel exploration, the mixed blessings of technology and the plague of nature-destroying overpopulation.

Throughout this adventure-rich time Jack and Stephen bond in a friendship based on mutual respect and loyalty. They complement each other in different spheres of their expert knowledge and, in the lulls between their duties and the inevitable wartime battles, they relax by playing duets together – Jack on the violin and Stephen on the cello. In fact, one product of the small industry spawned by O'Brian's imagination includes a CD of the music they played as they sailed around the world.[2]

## THE BACKGROUND OF THE AUBREY-MATURIN ADVENTURES

From the early 18th century to the middle of the 20th century, the British Navy was the largest and the most powerful seafaring force in the world, playing a key role in establishing the British Empire as the dominant world power of that era. Modern methods of financing by the government enabled this expansion of the navy. In the early 18th century, during naval operations in the War of the Spanish Succession, the British Navy captured Gibraltar (1704) and Port Mahon (1708). During the Napoleonic Wars, the Royal Navy dominated the navies of all its adversaries after defeating the numerically larger combined French and Spanish fleets at the Battle of Trafalgar on October 21, 1805. Subsequently, the navy patrolled the oceans in search of armed foes and looted their cargo ships. The years after Trafalgar saw increasing tension between Britain and the United States, caused by conflicting trade interests and the actions of the Royal Navy while enforcing a ban on the slave trade. In 1812 the United States declared war on the United Kingdom and invaded Canada. Throughout this period British naval vessels acted to suppress piracy, continued to map the world and made scientific observations.

O'Brian was a meticulous researcher and the descriptions of naval battles and other adventures in the novels are usually derived from the archives of the Royal Navy.

O'Brian's life is almost as interesting as that of his heroes, though in an entirely different manner. Born Richard Patrick Russ in Buckinghamshire, England in 1914, he published several well-respected works as a young man under that name. But in 1945, after collaborating with Mary Tolstoy on his *A Book of Voyages* in the early 1940s, she divorced Count Dmitri Tolstoy and Russ abandoned his wife and two children. They married in July, and in August he changed his name to Patrick O'Brian.[3] *Voyages* was always his favorite work because it brought them together, and her loss in 1998, nearly two years before O'Brian died, was "a tremendous blow."[4] In the 1950s he published two novels, *The Golden Ocean* and *The Unknown Shore*, based on Captain (later Admiral) George Anson's circumnavigation of the globe from 1740 to 1743, creating the characters Jack Byron and Tobias Barrow, antecedents of Maturin and Aubrey. But while Aubrey and Maturin sailed the globe pursuing Napoleon's fleet and often overpowering much larger enemy ships, O'Brian lived as a recluse in the small French village of Collioure, where he wrote by hand the Aubrey-Maturin series, as well as respected biographies of Pablo Picasso and Sir Joseph Banks, the famous English naturalist and botanist.

## MATURIN'S ORIGIN AND EDUCATION

Stephen Maturin is a son of an Irish officer and an aristocratic lady from Catalonia. His more distant antecedents, however, are not revealed. Jack Aubrey knows that Maturin owns a good piece of land in Catalonia with a tumbledown castle on it and that he is extremely frugal, except when it comes to books.

He is portrayed as a small, dark, white-faced individual in a rusty black coat. He is of indeterminate age, with a face that does not give anything away, but under this unassuming exterior dwells a very erudite and intelligent man with a remarkably good understanding of human nature. As a physician he is endowed with both surgical dexterity and diagnostic perspicacity. He is a musician and music lover, a competent zoologist, a botanist and a keen observer of other natural phenomena.

In a companion volume to O'Brian's novels called *A Sea of Words*, one of the co-authors, J.W. Estes, speculates that Maturin was probably born in the 1770s and was therefore about 30 when he joined the Royal Navy as a physician/surgeon.[5] This designation is significant because physicians were university trained and rated higher in the medical hierarchy than non-physician surgeons, who were considered craftsmen, although they ranked above apothecaries and assistants. In fact, the barber-surgeons, who had been very powerful in England and controlled the Company of Barber-Surgeons between about 1540 and 1745, were later pushed out by defecting surgeons, who in turn established the Company of Surgeons, which became The Royal College of Surgeons in 1800.[6]

O'Brian does not reveal where Maturin was trained but, according to Estes,[7] he received his premedical education at Trinity College in Dublin and studied medicine in France, claiming to have dissected with Guillaume Dupuytren (1777–1835), a noted French physician.

Stephen, whose loathing of Napoleon's imperial tyranny overrides his Irishman's natural antipathy for England, is actually an English spy, delivering periodic intelligence to a high-ranking government officer, Sir Joseph Blaine, with whom he shares an interest in the natural sciences.

> "Something of a polyglot – he is an accomplished linguist with a way of suiting his train of thought to the language that matched it best – Catalan, English, French, Castilian came to him as naturally as breathing, without preference, except for subject."[8]

When in India with H.M.S. *Surprise*, Maturin added Urdu to the linguistic center of his brain.

## MEDICAL TREATMENT

O'Brian equips Dr. Maturin with the totality of medical knowledge and the full medicinal armamentarium available at the beginning of the 19th century. At that time there was an understanding of the benefits derived from benign interventions, such as diet, exercise, rest, baths and massage, but there was also the wide application of bloodletting, cupping, blistering, sweating, emetics, purges, enemas and fumigation. Such procedures stemmed from the ancient belief that diseases were caused by an accumulation of noxious toxins and bad humors.

As to useful drugs, there was quinine for malaria, digitalis for heart failure, colchicine for gout and opium for pain and diarrhea. Of uncertain value were the widespread use of arsenic for nearly everything and antimony for fever and parasites. A variety of herbs, leaves, barks and roots applied in the form of powders, pills, extracts, infusions and decocta (boiling down to essence) was mostly of no value or even harmful. Indeed, among better-educated physicians, particularly of the French school, there was skepticism whether strong measures and drugs were helpful. They were prepared to allow diseases to take their own course. Maturin recognizes this. He observes that "medicine of his day could do very little and surgery less. He could purge patients, bleed or worm them, set their broken legs or take them off, and that was very nearly all." What, he asks, could Hippocrates, Galen, Rhazes, Blane or Trotter do for carcinoma, lupus, sarcoma? (Rhazes (AD 860–930) was a famous Arab physician who wrote brilliant descriptions of smallpox and measles; Gilbert Blane and Thomas Trotter were authors of textbooks on naval surgery.)[9]

At the same time, Maturin relies heavily in his practice on bleeding, cathartics, exceptionally bitter drafts and tonics, and he is an advocate of purging. For example, when he is called to consult on the condition of Lord Clonfort, captain of one of the ships under Commodore Aubrey's command, and finds him doubled up with abdominal pain, he diagnoses "colonic spasm" and prescribes a concoction of 20 minims of *Helleborus niger* with 40 drops of thebaic tincture and 60 of antimonial wine, accompanied with a little Armenian bole, all of which is to have the effect of "enemata." He finds this effective and his hardy patients know that they have been purged at both ends. Once he even uses an emetic to make a sailor vomit a swallowed musket ball.

When Spanish influenza breaks out on one of Aubrey's ships, Maturin doses the crew with a

> comfortable little prophylactic – undoubtedly physics, such as calomel (mercury chloride), jalap (exogonium purga from Mexico), medicinal rhubarb, castor oil, or cremor tartar (sodium potassium tartrate), a strong cathartic that was a major ingredient in Maturin's black draught, as well as tartar emetic (antimony potassium tartrate) and ipecac.[10]

After Jack's ship is boarded and taken by a privateer – one of the few such incidents in Aubrey's otherwise conquering career – Stephen gives this draft to the wounded Jack, who begins to regain consciousness after some hours in coma.[11]

The chief diseases that sailors suffer during long sea voyages are bad colds (known as catarrhs), influenza, tuberculosis (consumption) and pneumonia. Other afflictions include malaria, dysentery and bilious fever, a liver condition that produces jaundice (hepatitis). Stephen employs cinchona (Peruvian bark) to treat malaria. Syphilis and gonorrhea are common following any shore leave and, like his contemporaries, he uses mercuric chloride in the form of his famous "blue pill" and unguents (ointments) to treat both conditions, while forbidding all forms of alcohol to sailors recovering from venereal diseases.[12]

Maturin keeps up with medical advances. He knows that a dog bite can cause hydrophobia (rabies) and that mumps in adult men can cause sterility, and he is familiar with disorders that have their origin in the mind – false pregnancies, hysterias, palpitations, dyspepsias, eczema and some forms of impotence.

Naval doctors in those days had to procure their own supplies. Just as Captain Aubrey has to pay for repairs at shipyards where he takes refuge after his naval engagements, so Maturin must purchase his own drugs, using some of his share of the ships' prize money to buy such products as asafetida, castoreum and other substances that make his medicines thoroughly revolting in taste, smell and texture.

## MATURIN'S REFLECTIONS

To amplify the image of an all-around man, O'Brian makes Stephen something of a philosopher. While contemplating the hierarchy among British naval officers he muses that there is a spread of good qualities in the character of seamen with an inversion of rank, with amiable characteristics found in abundance among midshipmen and decreasing among lieutenants, captains and admirals. In a conversation with his colleague, Dr. McAdam, he observes that psychosomatic conditions do not exist aboard ship.

> "However, when sailors leave their natural environment, they are subject to a grievous list of infirmities – pox, drunkenness, over-eating which destroys the liver, anxiety, hypochondria, melancholia, delicate stomachs, weight loss, urine retention, black stools."[13]

Discussing the relationship between mind and body, McAdam suggests that one reason for the lack of mental illness in common sailors is that they are simply too busy to imagine non-existent problems.

## PREVENTIVE MEDICINE

Stephen is an unusual doctor for any age in that he is aware of the beneficial as well as the baneful effects of nutrition. He knows that scurvy will attack any ship lacking supplies of citrus fruit and vegetables. When several sick sailors from another vessel that had been at sea for months come aboard the *Surprise*, he whips out his copy of Blane's *Diseases of Seamen* and diagnoses scurvy by noting the men's "weakness, diffuse muscular pain, petechiae [minute hemorrhage in the skin or in a mucus or serous membrane], tender gums and ill breath."[14] When he thinks Aubrey's wife, Sophie, is too thin he recommends porter (a beer) with dinner. And he is constantly after Jack Aubrey to eat less and lose weight, warning him that he is digging his grave with his teeth. Stephen treats Aubrey's sorrow over an unhappy love affair before his marriage to Sophie with a curious diet of demulcent barley water and thin gruel, while forbidding beef, mutton and alcohol. (What he really seems to be doing is treating Jack's incipient obesity with a pre-Weight-Watcher's solution to the natural beefiness of ample and ruddy Englishmen.) But he also prescribes a thin watery gruel and no red meat for an officer with a shoulder injury, which only shows that the limited remedies of the early 19th century had to be spread in many directions. Stephen is never shy with nutritional advice for Jack Aubrey. He chastises Jack for helping himself to four portions of duck, which he calls "a melancholy meat"[15], and reminds him that the sauce in which it was marinated and cooked contains fat in abundance and should be absolutely forbidden to someone who is already as ample as Jack Aubrey. Never afraid to frighten his patients, Stephen mentions that apoplexy hides in this sort of dish and reminds Jack that he tried numerous times to catch his eye and discourage his appetite but to no avail, as Jack paid no heed to his efforts.

Maturin's reputation in the British Navy is one of scientific eminence. No less a person than the Physician of the Fleet observed that Maturin's book, *Tar-Water Reconsidered*, should be in every naval surgeon's chest. His library contains several widely read textbooks on a variety of medical and surgical subjects. He treats members of the nobility and admirals successfully. He diagnoses illness from the pulse, breathing, appearance of the tongue, stool and urine, and he recommends a quart of porter after blood loss but no wine, beef, mutton or sex, only fish, chicken, rabbits and, before retiring, a glass or two of cold negus (a combination of wine, hot water, sugar, nutmeg and lemon, named for Colonel Francis Negus, the British officer who invented it in the early 18th century) as well as physic and bolus (a mass of food or drugs, ready to be swallowed.)[16]

His wide-ranging skills even include delivering babies when they unfortunately arrive aboard ship to women either supposed or not supposed to be there. And in one instance he circumcises an intelligence agent who wishes to pass for a Jew, later meeting the gentleman, who acknowledges that "he feared it would never be quite the member it was."[17]

## HEROIC MEASURES

In *Master and Commander*, Stephen resuscitates a drowning victim, whose heart has stopped, with the following procedure. First he has him strung up by the heels and swings him back and forth two or three times to empty his lungs of water; then he bleeds him behind the ears; next, he lights a cigar and draws the smoke into a bellows, thrusting the nozzle of the bellows into the patient's nose and, while his assistant holds his mouth and other nostril closed, blows smoke into his lungs, all the while swinging his body so that "now his bowels pressed upon his diaphragm and now they did not. The result – gasps, choking, coughing and return to life."[18] O'Brian must have consulted a physician who told him that the two essential ingredients in resuscitating a drowned person are cough to empty the lungs of water and chest compression to maintain blood circulation, so that theoretically it could have worked. And while unorthodox to us, it was apparently not unknown in the 18th century. In *Revolutionary Medicine*, Dr. C. Keith Wilbur describes and illustrates two methods of removing water from the lungs of drowning victims: one was to put the man over a wooden barrel and roll him back and forth to compress the chest and force the water out; the second was to hang him upside down from a tree branch, put pressure on the chest and then remove it, allowing inspiration to occur. Wilbur, a medical historian, observes: "Inversion of the body was apparently successful."[19]

Maturin has uncommon surgical skills. He uses a trephine – a crown saw for removing a circular disk of bone from the skull – to treat a depressed skull fracture in one of the early novels, amputates limbs when necessary and sutures wounds. He does a suprapubic cystotomy to relieve urinary retention and sews on a severed ear.

But surely the most remarkable (and least believable) surgical procedure takes place in Calcutta while Aubrey's current command, the H.M.S. *Surprise*, is being repaired after a major battle. Stephen looks up Diana Villers, whom he has loved from a distance for years, and ends up in a duel while protecting her honor. He is wounded, taking a flattened and deflected bullet right under the pericardium. Refusing military surgeons and hospital, he decides to remove the bullet himself with Aubrey and McAlister, Stephen's aide, assisting. Here O'Brian boldly oversteps the boundaries of probability by having them hoist him on a stack of several chests and placing a mirror opposite him so that he can view the operative field and the assembled surgical instruments – crowbills, retractors, a toothed demi-lune (a crescent-shaped object) – which are placed within reach on a table. Without a word about analgesia or proper means to control bleeding beyond the application of pressure, Stephen slashes open his chest and instructs Jack and McAlister to retract the ribs using the square retractor and raise them up far enough so that McAlister can snip the cartilage. By this time Jack Aubrey is as white as the sheets below Stephen's body as he listens to Stephen's continual orders and the clash of medical instruments, and as he watches McAlister constantly swabbing up blood, aware all at once of the cruel force of injury that was greater than anything he had ever imagined or experienced in battle. The obliging bullet had settled under the pericardium, apparently and amazingly without injuring the heart. The procedure seems to go on and on as Stephen orders Aubrey to keep a steady downward pressure. Asking abruptly for the davier (forceps), ordering more swabbing and pressure, to Aubrey's amazement Stephen draws in a deep breath and arches his back. Without a cry of pain, with only a grunt, Stephen removes the bullet. Seemingly unperturbed, he asks whether the flattened bullet is whole. "Whole, sir, by God, quite whole. Not a morsel left."[20] Then, after the application of absorbent cotton on the raw, exposed tissue, Stephen tells McAlister to sew up the wound. Jack, looking at his watch, sees that the whole procedure, which had seemed to go on for hours, actually took only 23 minutes.

Now it is perfectly clear from this dramatic but unlikely incident that Patrick O'Brian has fallen in love with his remarkable doctor and given him not only scientific and medical knowledge and skill but also extreme strength of character to be able to self-inflict so much pain without hardly a murmur, while any normal man would be screaming his head off. The reader should remain aware that, in this instance alone, he has been exposed to pure fantasy, as likely as if Stephen had acquired wings that made him able to float in the sky.

However brilliant Maturin is intellectually, the combination of his unassuming physical appearance and the absence of a fortune (until quite late in life) explains his lack of success with women. The unhappiness over his unrequited love of Diana Villers and her involvement with other men may be responsible for his addiction to laudanum and later to coca leaves, which he collects during a trek in the Andes. Diana, a cousin of Jack Aubrey's wife Sophie, is beautiful, daring, clever but penniless. Thus her marriage prospects are, at the beginning of these 20 novels, rather negligible, though they improve at the end. Her choices of men are governed mostly by the weight of their purses, and her somewhat scandalous adventures periodically enliven the novels. The most exciting episode takes place in *The Fortune of War* when Stephen, a prisoner of war in Boston, while arranging an escape for himself and Aubrey, is forced to kill two French agents in order to rescue Diana from her current lover, Johnson, a wealthy and unscrupulous businessman and American intelligence agent, who attempted unsuccessfully to turn Stephen into an American spy. O'Brian describes Diana as aware of men's belief in their own superiority and notes that men only dimly grasped her underlying strength and that they wondered about her expression of secret amusement, a sort of relish of something that she did not choose to share.

For all his success with patients and interesting specimen collections, Stephen is presented as a somewhat despondent man, lonely and seeking the love of a woman he cannot have. But in the later novels O'Brian relents: Stephen comes into possession of a fortune; he can marry Diana at last and they produce a remarkable daughter, Bridget. Perhaps this is the author's announcement that he believes worthy men like Dr. Maturin deserve to end well.

Obviously O'Brian has been carried away in his idealized portrayal of the multi-talented Stephen Maturin. Or has he? If you look at Maturin's contemporaries, O'Brian has fashioned a fictional doctor not far off the mark. Take the career of a slightly older physician, and we see similarities. William Withering (1741–99), who is best known for his discovery of digitalis, was far more than a clinical physician, although he was a very good one indeed, with the largest provincial practice in the city of Birmingham. His M.D. came from the respected University of Edinburgh, but he was also a botanist, mineralogist and student of natural history. He was a member of Birmingham's Lunar Society, where he hobnobbed with Joseph Priestly (discoverer of oxygen, nitrogen and ammonia, and inventor of carbonated beverages), Erasmus Darwin (grandfather of Charles and an early evolutionist), Josiah Wedgwood (whose porcelain has come down to us through the generations) and James Watt (who invented a more efficient steam engine, the pressure gauge and the double-action piston, while adding his name to the language forever in the form of watt and kilowatt).[21]

We have to acknowledge that the better class of English physician of this time was incredibly well educated in all the known natural sciences, a possibility that no longer exists with the information explosion in every field, which makes the existence today of a broadly educated humanist like those of the 18th or 19th centuries extremely unlikely.

## REFERENCES

1 O'Brian P. *Aubrey-Maturin* series. New York: WW Norton; 1960–1999:
*Master and Commander* 1969
*Post Captain* 1972
*HMS Surprise* 1973
*The Mauritius Command* 1977
*Desolation Island* 1978
*The Fortune of War* 1979
*The Surgeon's Mate* 1980
*The Ionian Mission* 1981
*Treason's Harbor* 1983
*The Far Side of the World* 1984
*The Reverse of the Medal* 1986
*The Letter of Marque* 1988
*The Thirteen-Gun Salute* 1989
*The Nutmeg of Consolation* 1991
*The Truelove* 1992 (*Clarissa Oakes* in Britain)

*The Wine-Dark Sea* 1993
*The Commodore* 1994
*The Yellow Admiral* 1996
*The Hundred Days* 1998
*Blue at the Mizzen* 1999

2  *Musical Evenings with the Captain by Philharmonia Virtuosi.* ESS.A.Y. Recordings; 1996.

3  O'Brian P. *A Book of Voyages.* London: Home & Van Thal; 1947.

4  Tolstoy N. *Patrick O'Brian: the making of a novelist.* London: Century; 2004.

5  King D, Estes JW, Hattendorf JB. *A Sea of Words.* 2nd ed. New York: Henry Holt and Company; 2000.

6  The Royal College of Surgeons of England. *History of the College.* Available at: www. rcseng.ac.uk/about/history

7  King, Estes, Hattendorf, op. cit.

8  O'Brian P. *HMS Surprise.* p. 16.

9  O'Brian P. *Surprise.* p. 119.

10  O'Brian P. *Post Captain.* p. 122.

11  Ibid., pp. 135–6.

12  Ibid., p. 297.

13  O'Brian P. *Post Captain.* pp. 99–100.

14  O'Brian P. *HMS Surprise.* p. 118.

15  Ibid., p. 278.

16  O'Brian P. *Post Captain.* pp. 387–8.

17  O'Brian P. *Fortune of War.* p. 20.

18  O'Brian P. *Master and Commander.* p. 286.

19  Wilbur CK. *Revolutionary Medicine: 1700–1800.* Old Saybrook: The Globe Pequat Press; 1980. p. 19.

20  O'Brian P. *HMS Surprise.* p. 353.

21  Birminghamuk.com. *Lunar Society.* Available at: www.birminghamuk.com/lunar society.htm

# CHAPTER 3

# Dr. Tertius Lydgate

## in *Middlemarch*

by George Eliot[1]

---

### Themes

- A remarkable woman writer and intellectual
- A real-life picture of provincial England in the 1830s, at the start of the Reform Movement
- Authentic review of medical practice
- The clash of ambition and reality

---

Mary Ann Evans was the fifth and youngest child of Robert Evans, a poor farmer whose cleverness and hard work advanced him to a position of land agent to the Newdigate family of Arbory Halls, a sumptuous estate with a large library available for intense exploration by the future George Eliot during her adolescence. In a biography of George Eliot (1819–80), Kathryn Hughes emphasized that Mary Ann, dubbed the "last Victorian" in the subtitle of her biography,[2] was born in the same year as the future Queen Victoria, marking the time frame of her creative writing.

Her early years spent in the Griff farmhouse exposed her to the chores and rhythm of agricultural life, memories of which played a prominent role in some of her future novels. A major problem at this time was the lack of any viable relationship with her mother, a woman incapable of giving her youngest child the love she craved, and who died at an early age. The story of how a girl born into a farming class ascended to become one of the leading literary and intellectual figures of the day reveals the confluence of the diverse talents nourishing her creativity. At all stages of her life she was able to commit to memory the visual images of her surroundings and the diversity of human speech patterns and vocabularies peculiar to regions and the various levels of education, while at the same time observing human interactions and social events. In her reading she strived to absorb the essence of human culture within a wide range of subjects, from mathematics, physics and biology to philosophy, religion, music (she was a gifted pianist) and literature, which, thanks to her knowledge of several foreign languages, she could read in the original. This background explains her facility in writing elegantly structured letters, essays, book reviews and translations of scientific and literary works.

During her adolescence and up to the age of 21 she was a strict, devout evangelical Anglican, but she abruptly distanced herself from the character of the authentic Christian, probably after she diversified her reading from works dedicated exclusively to God to the romantic poets and scientific works that paved the way to Darwin's questioning of Creation. When, at this time, the family moved to Coventry, her refusal as a free-thinker to accompany her father to church initiated a difficult period, which she later called a "holy war" and which forced her to take refuge in nearby Rosehill, the home of the equally free-minded young silk manufacturer Charles Bray, his wife Cara, and Cara's sister, Sara Hennell. She forged a life-long friendship with all of them. In the Bray's house she met many intellectuals, including the socialist Robert Owen, the philosopher Herbert Spencer and the American poet Ralph Waldo Emerson. Her friends describe her as a young woman falling in love with every man or woman igniting her intellectual curiosity, but suffering from her image as an ugly woman – tall, gawky, with a long nose, thick lips and a large head that was sometimes compared to a horse. Being of marriageable age, she observed in her surroundings the failures of this institution among incompatible partners.

In 1851 and 1852 Mary Ann entered the household of John Chapman in London. The young, dashing Chapman edited the *Westminster Review*, a leading intellectual quarterly of the day. Recognizing Mary Ann's talent, the editor assigned to her the preparation of essays and book reviews for the journal, which sharpened her writing skills. She apparently had a brief affair with Chapman, whom many thought was the model for Tertius Lydgate, the doctor hero of *Middlemarch*, before she met George Henry Lewes – a writer, philosopher and naturalist, with whom she eloped to Germany. This man, apparently as ugly as Mary Ann, was a passionate and versatile intellectual with an atheistic upbringing, in whom Mary Ann encountered a partner matching her superior intellect. Unfortunately Lewes was not free to marry her, because he was already married, although separated from his wife, who, in addition to the three sons fathered by Lewes, had three more with Thornton Hunt, her lover, during the time she was still married to Lewes. By adopting Hunt's children to relieve his wife's financial straits, Lewes forfeited the right to a divorce. The status of living with a married man initially narrowed the range of Evans' social contacts, but after the appearance of her novels, her mass popularity, often reaching adoration, broke all social barriers for the cultural elite seeking contact with Marian Lewes, as she preferred to be called. The pen name George Eliot reflects her wish to distance herself from the majority of contemporary female writers, whom she satirized in an essay written in 1856 called *Silly Novels by Lady Novelists.*[3] She objected to their inept fiction featuring romances between scions of the titled aristocracy while being unable to describe actual life. More cogent reasons for a male pseudonym were her initial, and never completely dispelled, fear of a disapproving critique, and her perceived status as a cast-out woman.

The unshakable liaison between Mary Ann Evans and George Henry Lewes, based on physical attraction and intellectual kinship, was mutually gratifying. He nudged her to write and then publish her works after they passed his critical assessment. She reciprocated by her interest in his writings, as evidenced by her ability to complete his work *Problems of Life and Mind* after his death.

Between 1858 and 1876 George Eliot published nine highly regarded and avidly read novels, elevating her to celebrity status and making her wealthy. Unlike the characters in the books of her contemporary Charles Dickens, her heroes and heroines could not be dubbed as wholly evil or wholly decent, as there are some redeeming qualities in the villains and some flaws in the noble characters. Also there are no conspicuous rewards for decency. Her heroes may struggle against the oppressive circumstances within small-minded communities, but in the course of their lives they discover that the way to moral growth is reconciliation. Her characters were well understood by contemporary readers because they dealt with the "concerns of intellectual Victorians, how to balance the rights of the individual with the needs of others."[4] She strongly believed that fiction should not be didactic but should express philosophical ideas as they reveal themselves in the actions of her heroes and that writing should not be exclusively preachy or lapse into a form of rigid diagrams. Socially she was conservative, fearing to give voting rights to the working class or to women lacking moral and social education. She was also concerned about the impact of the hurried pace of modern life, which was threatening the sense of community in pre-industrial Britain.

Her self-education never ceased. In her last major novel, *Daniel Deronda*, she introduced several Jewish characters, prompting her to learn Hebrew and evoke the vision of a Jewish state in Palestine 20 years before the concept of Zionism emerged in Theodor Herzel's book. After Dickens and Thackeray died and Trollope was past his peak, George Eliot was the country's greatest novelist. Two years after Lewes' death, she married in a church ceremony a wealthy friend, John Cross, 20 years her junior. He became her earliest biographer, following her death from kidney failure only 10 months after the wedding.

The popularity of George Eliot's novels waned with time, occasionally resurging when produced by Masterpiece Theater and other film makers. Her place in the pantheon of great English writers, however, is assured as the truest literary chronicler of the historical period she portrayed in the immaculate prose of her novels.


## THE NOVEL

*Middlemarch* is the title of her sprawling Victorian novel, which appeared in eight parts between 1869 and 1872, and is the name of a thriving market town in the Midlands. Its inhabitants work in a silk factory and in the surrounding agricultural estates owned by the county gentry. The novel opens in 1829, revealing a social and political provincial life in agitation over the events leading up to the 1832 Great Reform Act. This Act produced the first child labor laws in the textile industry, limiting children between the ages of 13 to 18 to 12-hour work days and those between eight and 13 to six and a half hours of work a day. The book reveals the relationship between town and country and shows how the society works. From a multitude of memorable characters involved in complex plots and sub-plots in the novel, the two principal heroes are the 19-year-old niece of a widowed landowner, Dorothea Brooke, and the 27-year-old doctor, Tertius Lydgate. Their stories run in parallel but intersect occasionally, with both characters having in common a desire to improve the lot of the local people and both becoming victims of disastrous marriages. Dorothea is clever and intelligent but expects more wisdom and knowledge in the company of an older man, without realizing that her chosen husband, the clergyman Casaubon, is a rigid, humorless pedant paralyzed by fear of failure and stuck hopelessly in a futile attempt to write his planned life-work, *The Key to All Mythologies.*

The models for Dorothea were abundant in the writer's life experience and her own self-knowledge, but with Lydgate she needed to understand the practice of medicine. Her brother-in-law exemplified a physician settled in a marriage with nine children, who falls into debt and bankruptcy and is unable to maintain a proper lifestyle, earning a meager income from a practice with largely impecunious patients in a small town. To describe a hospital she made a two-day visit to Leeds Infirmary. From Lewes' days as a medical student she learned about anatomy and the pathology of prevalent illnesses, including typhoid and cholera. She read extensively about the organization and practice of provincial hospitals and all aspects of the developments in medicine.

The handsome Lydgate arriving in this provincial town is a gentleman by birth, with

> a voice habitually deep and sonorous yet capable of becoming very low and gentle at the right moment. About his ordinary bearing there was a certain fling, a fearless expectation of success, a confidence in his own powers and integrity much fortified by contempt for petty obstacles or seductions of which he had no experience.[5]

He had qualified in medicine at the prestigious universities of Edinburgh and Paris. Armed with stethoscope, microscope and tools for dissection of cadavers, he feels superior to the resident doctors of an older vintage and is ready to combine the modern practice of general medicine with meaningful research. His role model is Edward Jenner (1749–1823), a practitioner whose keen observation of milkmaids with cowpox led to the discovery of the small-pox vaccine. His other admired giants of medicine include François Bichat (1771–1802), a pioneer in anatomical pathology, René Laennec (1781–1826), inventor of the stethoscope, and Pierre Louis (1787–1872), an expert on typhoid fever who established the importance of statistics in medical research.

Lydgate loves medicine because it provides "the most perfect interchange between science and art; offering the most direct alliance between intellectual conquest and the common good." In fact, he is eager to do "good small work for Middlemarch and great work for the world."[6] Not unexpectedly, both elude him.

He is, however, an astute physician. From Casaubon's complaints he recognizes angina pectoris and knows its propensity to sudden cardiac death, which he explains to both Dorothea and Casaubon. This is an astonishing observation in 1830. Equally amazing is that he attributes Casaubon's angina to coronary artery disease, which he calls "fatty degeneration of the heart," crediting the work of Laennec. Although coronary artery disease was an entity unknown to the average general practitioner in the English provinces at this time, Eliot must have read Laennec's work as well as Caleb Parry's 1799 paper that connected angina and coronary artery disease. In fact, it seems that Eliot appropriated every medical advance of the period and gave them all to her brilliant doctor.

Lydgate understands the ineffectiveness of many prescribed drugs and equally abhors the concepts of the "strengtheners," who use such remedies as port wine and bark to add to their patient's substance, and the "lowerers," who either remove blood through cupping or order physic, which clears the system of noxious elements. Instead, when useful remedies are not available, he prefers to have the disease run its own course. However, by refusing to conform to the established practice of physicians procuring their drugs from the pharmacist and selling them to patients at a profit, he antagonizes both the pharmacist and the doctors. He also annoys the wealthy banker, perhaps the one person in town who could afford and was willing to build him his dream "fever hospital," where he imagines himself studying the causes of infectious diseases by examining cadavers, another reason for the distrust of his colleagues, who are averse to autopsies. But his biggest mistake is to let himself be trapped into a marriage with Rosamund Vincy, the pretty daughter of the town's mayor.

Lydgate, while a student in Paris, had become enamored of a beautiful actress. After stabbing her husband to death on stage during a play in which she was required only to pretend to do so, she claimed it was an accident and was not prosecuted. Lydgate chased her to Lyon and was only dissuaded from his offer of marriage after she confessed she did it on purpose. She told him he was a good man but claimed she did not like husbands and would never remarry. Though determined not to engage in such folly again, and certainly not to marry for at least five years because he could not afford a wife, Lydgate is nonetheless beguiled by Rosamund, who sets her mind on marrying him because he is a baronet, which fits her ambition to rise among the gentry and never consort with anyone who is "common." Rosie is not an unscrupulous schemer but a typical young woman raised for a proper marriage. She has no intellectual interests but is accomplished in those things that young women of her time were supposed to master – music (she plays the piano and sings well), clothes (lots of ruffles, silks, satins, headdresses), art (she draws and paints) and gossip (the major recreation of this pre-electronic communication era). For most young suitors she would be an excellent choice, but Lydgate needs a partner who understands his mind and his ideas and supports his ambition. And this is not the case. Trying to meet her expensive living standards, he is ruined financially; he is dispirited and forced to abandon his dreams of a "fever hospital," even when Dorothea offers the financial help which could have resurrected his project. He considers himself a failure because he had not done what he meant to do. At the end of the novel he muses sadly:

> Only those who know the supremacy of the intellectual life – the life which has a seed of ennobling thought and purpose within it – can understand the grief of one who falls from that serene activity into this absorbing soul-wasting struggle with worldly annoyances.[7]

Instead he becomes a society doctor in London, supported by rich patients. Even in this milieu he manages to produce a treatise on gout. He sires children and lives in comfort but dies at age 50. Objectively, this is far from an utterly failed life. Yet this is his own epitaph: "I had some ambition. I meant everything to be different with me. I thought I had more strength and mastery. But the most terrible obstacles are such as nobody can see except oneself."[8]

Dorothea also escapes misery. True to Lydgate's prediction, Casaubon dies from a heart attack and, after a proper mourning period, she is free to reciprocate the love of a penniless but charming journalist, a distant cousin of Casaubon, whom she earlier encountered in a museum in Florence. They marry and move to London, where they have two children and he becomes a Member of Parliament.

For a contemporary physician, the life of Lydgate offers no relevant lessons. The income of physicians in developed countries today comes largely from the insured population and not from assorted wealthy clients. The dream of making an important scientific discovery while in full-time private practice, such as the one made by Jenner, has little chance of fulfillment. Not far from realism, however, is the image of a young graduate of a good training program who comes to town with more knowledge than is available to the established old-timers, but today such a physician is likely to join an established group practice rather than isolate himself in a solo practice. Lydgate may be the best-educated physician in Middlemarch, but he is arrogant, impulsive and intolerant of human foibles. Such characters are usually punished by society, and Lydgate's punishment is his loss of idealism. However, because George Eliot provides a remarkably accurate picture of medical practice in 1830s England, and does so with an absorbing plot and excellent prose, this novel is definitely worth reading.

## REFERENCES

1 Eliot G (1871–72). *Middlemarch*. New York: Barnes and Noble Classics; 2003.
2 Hughes K. *George Eliot: the last Victorian*. New York: Cooper Square Press; 2001.
3 Ibid., p. 177.
4 Ibid., p. 303.
5 Eliot, op. cit., p. 152.
6 Ibid., p. 174.
7 Ibid., p. 793.
8 Ibid., p. 821.

**PART TWO**

# Idealistic doctors

# CHAPTER 4

# Dr. Martin Arrowsmith

## in *Arrowsmith*

### by Sinclair Lewis[1]

---

### Themes

- Medical practice and public health
- Medical education in the United States in the early 20th century
- Greed and ignorance among physicians
- Ethics in medical research

---

Sinclair Lewis (1885–1951) was 40 years old when he published *Arrowsmith* in 1925. It is a novel which portrays the best and worst aspects of American medicine in the first quarter of the 20th century. The son of a country doctor in Minnesota, whose brother Claude was a surgeon, Sinclair Lewis had apparently thought about a career in medicine while a student at Yale. In the Afterword of the book, Mark Schorer, Lewis' biographer, points out that, after the social criticism and satire in *Main Street* and *Babbitt*, Lewis had an impulse to write a heroic novel and medicine was a logical choice.[2] From his friend Paul DeKruif, then a young bacteriologist, he learned a great deal about medical science and research.[3]

The tall, unathletic, gangly third son of a strict father, Sinclair Lewis was a sort of odd man out, with few friends during his public school years in Sauk Centre, Minnesota, at Oberlin Academy and at Yale. He dropped out of college for a year to work at Helicon Hall, Upton Sinclair's utopian community in New Jersey, and to travel to Panama, finally graduating in 1908. He described his university career as undistinguished, except for contributions of stories to the *Yale Literary Magazine*. In his autobiography for the Nobel Committee, he recalled these stories as "reeking with a banal romanticism,"[4] surely not an accurate herald of the mature author known for portraying ordinary Americans on the typical main streets of the Midwest. He published a string of unsuccessful novels between 1914 and 1919, claiming, "I lacked sense enough to see that after five failures, I was foolish to continue writing."[5] It was a lucky bit of foolishness because *Main Street*, which came out in 1920, was, according to Schorer, "the most sensational event in twentieth-century American publishing history," selling initially 180,000 copies and a total of two million within the next few years.[6] Lewis went on to write *Elmer Gantry*, *Dodsworth* and, in 1935, *It Can't Happen Here*, which speculated about the possible election of a fascist U.S. President. In all, he published 25 novels between 1912 and his death from alcoholism in 1951.

## THE NOVEL

Martin Arrowsmith is a new type of hero in American fiction, reflecting the demands, challenges and nobility of the medical profession. When the action begins in 1904, Martin is a 21-year-old arts and science major in his junior year at the University of Winnemac in the mythological state of the same name (bordered by Michigan, Ohio, Illinois and Indiana), preparing for medical school. He is pale, has smooth black hair and is "a respectable runner, a fair basketball center and a savage hockey player."[7]

### Love life – personal

Once in medical school Arrowsmith feels himself far superior to his classmates due to his interest in research, though he is totally ignorant of literature, painting or music. He quickly reconnects with Madeline Fox, a girl he knew in college, a high-spirited and handsome tennis-playing showoff, socially ambitious and determined, a dabbler in culture and a Ph.D. candidate in the Department of English, where she admires Hardy, Meredith, Howells and Thackeray, and where she is eventually told she doesn't have the stuff (curiosity, intelligence?) to attain such glorified academic heights. Martin woos her while her battleaxe of a mother stands guard, and he finally proposes when he finds her unhappy at the discovery of her blocked career aspirations, even though he has years of schooling and training ahead of him. Mama approves, however, and the couple settles for a commitment to a very long engagement.

Shortly he meets a very different type of a woman – the "girl-next-door." She is Leora Tozer from North Dakota, a probationary nurse at Zenith General Hospital, where Professor Gottlieb, Martin's mentor, has sent him to collect a blood sample from a patient with meningitis. Leora, scrubbing a floor, is delightfully fresh as he asks for directions to Ward D, and Martin, smitten, starts a second courtship, proposing in jig time. This collecting of fiancées is done without the slightest hint of passion, except for an occasional stolen kiss, as nice girls did not "put out" in those days. Leora is not really interested in nursing; she's here for the adventure and to get away from Wheatsylvania, where her father, Andrew Jackson Tozer, owns the bank, the creamery and a grain elevator, and where she has a bedridden great aunt who can presumably benefit from whatever nursing skills she acquires.

Puzzled by how to solve this overabundance of prospective brides, Martin invites both girls to luncheon at the Grand Hotel in Zenith to choose a wife. The haughty and elegant Madeline shows off her superiority and snobbishness toward the unsophisticated, innocent, loveable and charming farm girl, and when Martin confesses the true purpose of the lunch, Madeline indignantly stalks off, leaving Leora victorious on the field of matrimonial battle.

Martin visits Leora in Wheatsylvania, and finds her

> absurd in a huge coonskin coat. He must have looked a little mad as he stared at her from the vestibule, as he shivered with the wind. She lifted to him her two open hands, childish in red mittens. He ran down, he dropped his awkward bag on the platform and, unaware of the gaping furry farmers, they were lost in a kiss. Years after, in a tropic noon, he remembered the freshness of her wind cooled cheeks.[8]

The Tozers think Martin should finish medical school and start earning money before getting married. Martin and Leora want no part of this propriety and elope to the county seat, where they are legally joined together by a German Lutheran pastor. Her father, furious, refuses to let them sleep in the same bedroom; he sends his son Burt to patrol the hallway, and he chases Martin back to finish medical school. But Martin returns to Wheatsylvania to defy Tozer and collect Leora. They rent a room in Zenith and finally consummate their marriage. Leora begins to study stenography. She is pregnant, suffers from vicious vomiting, loses the baby at six months and cannot have more children, but the marriage endures.

## Love life – medicine

Martin has long been enraptured by medicine. As a young boy he helped Dr. Vickerson, the alcoholic physician in his home town, while reading through his copy of *Gray's Anatomy*. Once Martin is in medical school, Dr. Max Gottlieb, an immigrant German Jew and professor of microbiology, becomes his hero and mentor. Gottlieb was trained at Heidelberg but was not much interested in bandaging legs and looking at tongues. He admired Helmholtz, whose research in the physics of sound convinced Gottlieb that the medical sciences needed a quantitative methodology. Then Koch's discoveries drew him into microbiology and he worked in both Koch's and Pasteur's laboratories. Gottlieb understands that research is rigorous, methodical, undramatic, tedious and unappreciated. More than the fear of starvation, he hated researchers who rush into publication unprepared. Extremely uncompromising, publicity-shy and self-critical, Gottlieb is demanding of himself and others in the service of scientific truth.

Medical school is drudgery but Martin feels how it sets the students apart from ordinary folk; they use sawed-off skulls for ashtrays and hang a skeleton, bought on installment plan, in their bedroom. But the real joy is the laboratory, which mesmerizes Martin, who is in awe of

> the roaring Bunsen flames beneath the hot-air ovens, the steam from the Arnold sterilizers rolling to the rafters . . . the rows of test-tubes filled with watery serum and plugged with cotton singed to a coffee brown . . .[9]

Internship gives Martin a sense of power as he rides the ambulance to the scene of a fire, commands the driver and firemen, and gives out information to reporters. His black bag is his pass: policemen salute him and saloon keepers bow to him. Once he rescues a bank president from a dive and helps his family conceal the disgrace; another time he breaks into a hotel room to save a would-be suicide. He drinks rum with a Congressman who advocates prohibition, attends a policeman assaulted by strikers and strikers assaulted by police, assists at emergency operations, delivers a baby in a flooded tenement and even swims across a swollen river to save children marooned on a bobbing church pew.

Despite his fondness for research, he abandons Gottlieb and the laboratory for private practice in Leora's home town. Here Lewis gives us a realistic account of small-town practice. Martin pulls a raging infected tooth from his first patient's mouth with a dental forceps he acquired on the advice of the Dean – that a country doctor has to be "not only physician but dentist, yes, and priest, divorce lawyer, blacksmith, chauffeur, and road engineer."[10] Soon he faces a more serious challenge – a little girl very ill with diphtheria. He can either perform a tracheotomy or inject an antitoxin (discovered by Roux and Yersin around the end of the 19th century). Martin chooses the latter, takes a wild ride in the middle of the night to the next town, awakens the druggist to get the medicine, races back and finds the child barely alive. He injects the serum, but it is too late and the child dies. The parents blame the injection and Martin. Crushed, he swears he'll never practice medicine again but an older, wiser general practitioner gives him good advice – to consult a seasoned colleague in serious cases, not for advice, but to share the responsibility. Of course, this consultation comes at a price: this doc only charges "a little more than my regular fee, and it looks so well, talking the case over with an older man."[11]

There are glorious moments as well: one afternoon, returning from fishing, he passes a farmhouse from which a hysterical woman emerges screaming that her baby has swallowed a thimble and is choking to death. Martin has only a large jack-knife with him but, sharpening it on the farmer's oilstone, he uses the tea-kettle to boil water and sterilize the knife, makes an incision in the baby's throat, removes the object and saves the child's life. Every newspaper in the district carries the story and Martin is a local hero.

Probably he could have remained a successful country doctor if he had not needed different challenges. One comes in the form of an epidemic of blackleg among the cattle in the neighboring county, which evokes memories of his apprenticeship in bacteriology at medical school. Martin isolates the organism and prepares a vaccine, which stops the epidemic cold. But he is denounced by the county's veterinarians for intruding into their realm.

Soon he tires of the tedium and bickering with doctors in Wheatsylvania. He obtains a job in the Public Health Department of Nautilus, a much larger town. Here he starts working on a precipitation test for diagnosing syphilis, one that should be quicker and simpler than the Wasserman test. His boss is Dr. Pickerbaugh, a maverick and charlatan, whose preaching for cleanliness, hygiene and morality is aimed as a stepping stone to a political career while he neglects to attend to the important public health problems of his district. He is one of the editors of the *Midwest Medical Quarterly*, in which he publishes his scientific discoveries, among them the "germ" of epilepsy and two different "germs" of cancer. It usually takes Pickerbaugh two weeks to make a discovery, write it up and have it accepted in this journal.

Pickerbaugh is not Lewis' only caricature of a physician. Earlier in the novel Dr. Roscoe Geake, vice-president of the New Idea Medical Instrument and Furniture Company of Jersey City, lectures Martin's graduating medical school class, telling them that the world judges a man by the amount of cash he possesses. Wealth impresses patients, he says, allowing them to feel confident if the doctor requests proper compensation and has a luxurious office, preferably a mixture of the Aseptic and Tapestry Schools – the former featuring white-painted chairs with a single Japanese print against a gray wall, the latter using elegant furniture, cut-glass vases, potted palms, handsome pictures and bookcases jammed with expensively bound volumes of world literature.

No less cynical is a former classmate from medical school who is practicing in the same town and advises Martin to join the country club and take up golf as a way of attracting high-class patients. This greedy physician criticizes public health clinics because they create the habit in patients of getting free medical care rather than seeing private physicians, and he deplores Martin's treating the damn lazy pauper class in the city's free clinic. Another former classmate is an avaricious high-society surgeon, Dr. Angus Duer, whose luxurious offices and reception room in Chicago are like the drawing-room of an oil magnate.

While in Nautilus, Martin becomes absorbed in attempting to isolate a blood-destroying poison, hemolysin, produced by the streptococcus bacillus. The search soon becomes an obsession – to the point where he loses his job. But that's not the only reason for Martin's fall; he picked a fight with a slum landlady who had the right political connections. Before he is fired, however, he has been able to repeat his experiments and has started to develop a formula for the production of hemolysin, overcoming his rusty chemistry and inadequate mathematics. Slowly he assembles his results and has enough material for a scientific paper in the *Journal of Infectious Diseases*. Simultaneously he gets a notice that Professor Gottlieb, working at the McGurk Institute in New York City, has synthesized antibodies *in vitro*. Gottlieb sees Martin's paper and invites him to join him at the Institute because, "You know something of laboratory technique; you have heard about dese bacilli; you are not a good chemist, and mathematics – pfui! – most terrible! But you have curiosity and you are stubborn. You do not accept rules."[12]

At McGurk Martin feels he has come home. He is allowed to work on what interests him; soon research wipes out everything else in his life and he works night and day. One morning he isolates a new strain of staphylococcus and, after incubating it, obtains a good growth of bacteria within eight hours, but later that night he finds no sign of bacteria in the flask. He is amazed; it is as though the bacteria have committed suicide. He realizes he's hit on something.

Lewis describes Martin at this stage of his career:

> Now in Martin Arrowsmith there were no decorative heroisms, no genius for amours, no exotic wit, no edifyingly borne misfortunes. He presented neither picturesque elegance nor a moral message. He was full of hasty faults and of perverse honesty; a young man often unkindly, often impolite. But he had one gift: curiosity whereby he saw nothing as ordinary. Had he been an acceptable hero . . . he would have chucked the contents of the flask into the sink, avowed with pretty modesty, "Silly, I've made some error!" and gone on his way. But Martin, being Martin, walked prosaically up and down his laboratory, snarling, "Now there was some cause for that, and I'm going to find out what it was."[13]

To test possible reasons for the disappearance of staphylococci, he seeds with bacteria a series of flasks with varying conditions and sets them in the incubator at body temperature. Calmly he awaits the results. And he succeeds. He writes in his notes: "I have observed a principle, which I shall temporarily call the X Principle, in pus from a staphylococcus infection, which checks the growth of several strains of staphylococci, and which dissolves the staphylococci from the pus in question."[14] It turns out that, unknown to Martin, the discovery of bacteria-dissolving phage was published earlier by the French scientist d'Herrell. This robs Martin of his hour of glory, but he finds that the principle is applicable to the plague bacillus, which is killed by substance X, or phage, so that the infected rats are protected from death.

There is an epidemic of bubonic plague on the island of St. Hubert's in the Caribbean, and Martin travels there to test the efficacy of the phage. His mentor, Gustaf Sondelius, whom Lewis said was his favorite character, comes to help him. Sondelius is modeled on Dr. Alexis Karrel, the pioneer of organ transplantation and the first American to win the Nobel Prize in medicine and physiology. It was Karrel who roamed the world fighting epidemics and founding research institutes. Immediately Martin sees the dilemma he faces. If you want to establish the effectiveness of the phage, there must be a control group. This is a tough moral problem. Martin had promised Gottlieb that he would adhere to the experimental protocol, but watching people die this horrible death eats at him. He realizes that Gottlieb, in his secluded innocence, has no notion of what it means to experiment amid the hysteria of an epidemic.

Martin swears he will not yield to compassion by treating everybody with phage, which could deprive him of scientific evidence. Thus only half of patients in the district receive phage, amid the predictable outrage of the other half. People swear at him in the streets, throw stones at him, beg him for the medicine to cure the children. But even if shaken he must always keep the vision of Gottlieb before him to persist in treating with phage only every other person, while the rest of the treatment is the same for everyone. The plague affects the untreated half more heavily than the treated patients and it seems they are on the way to a successful conclusion when Leora dies and Martin breaks down. He turns the experiment over to a colleague, who proceeds with somewhat less rigid protocols that would not satisfy Martin and Gottlieb and the rest of the scientific world, so that a careful statistical analysis makes his conclusions less certain. Meanwhile Sondelius, who has worked side by side with Martin, is the first to recognize his own symptoms and immediately quarantines himself and dies. Martin, in his grief, gives the phage to everyone. Although he's a hero on St. Hubert's, he dreads going home to admit that he has thrown away his great chance – to prove unequivocally that it is possible to eliminate plague worldwide by this method.

Back in New York, Martin is lionized and appointed to head his own department. He marries Joyce Lanyon, a rich socialite, who tries to drag him into her milieu. They have a child. But Martin shuns the luxurious life at home and in the Institute, preferring to pursue his research with Terry Wickett, the one true uncompromising scientist at McGurk now that Gottlieb has retired. They find a cure for pneumonia but refuse to publish prematurely, despite pressure from the Institute. Wickett stomps off to Vermont, where he sets up a laboratory to pursue pure science. Martin divorces his wife and joins him. Terry had discovered that certain quinine derivatives decompose into products toxic to bacteria while being only mildly harmful to the body. Now they must determine whether the quinine derivatives act by attaching themselves to the bacteria or by changing the immune system.

Here Lewis leaves Martin, who has become an accomplished scientist with his mathematics and chemistry as sound as Terry's. He is indifferent to publicity and comfort, ready to use his fanatical energy to test a slew of hypotheses. Martin suddenly understands how to cherish his freedom. He believes he will yet determine the essential nature of phage and sees ahead of him numerous inquiries into chemotherapy and immunity, indeed "enough adventures to keep him busy for decades."[15]

## HOW PERTINENT ARE MARTIN ARROWSMITH'S EXPERIENCES TO THE CONTEMPORARY MEDICAL SCENE AND TO MEDICAL RESEARCH?

The initiation into the profession by rigor and drudgery, and the requirement to commit to memory the near limitless material in medical school and during internship has changed little with time. Also, the hectic pace of private practice, initially needed to pay off education-related debts, and later to maintain sufficient income to cover costly overhead, may leave a physician like Martin oblivious to the pleasures of literature, art and music. The triumphs and debacles when dealing with patients, the social climbing, the commercialization, the greed, the envy and the occasional incompetence – imbedded in human nature and inherent in the profession – are as prevalent today as they were in the past. Medical science in America, however, is far less deplorable today than in Martin's time, when his two role models in research were Europeans, one a German immigrant bacteriologist and the other a Swedish biologist.

Martin's research career, propelled largely by self-education without formal training, would be improbable today. Even more improbable would be the accomplishment of productive scientific work in a rustic laboratory on a farm in Vermont without a connection to an academic institution and grant support.

## MARTIN'S IDEALISM

Martin Arrowsmith emerges as a scientific truth-seeker and an uncompromising idealist whose integrity propels him to make a correct moral choice at each crossroad of his tortuous professional career. As a small-town practitioner he tries vainly to save the little girl with diphtheria, even though he has been called in too late to succeed; he loses his job in Nautilus because he offends the greedy slum proprietor with political connections and because his innate curiosity drives him to set up an original research project. He tries hard to stay the scientific course on St. Hubert's but yields to compassion by giving phage to everyone after losing Leora. At McGurk, although tempted by comfortable security, he abandons it to pursue pure unglamorous science under more spartan conditions. Martin is admirable and intensely human. More important, he is believable because of the character imperfections Lewis mixes with his strong and endearing assets.

But the scenario of medical science pictured in this novel is probably too fictional to inspire the young scientists of today's generation. Moreover, the drama on the island is not realistic, because experiments of this type are conducted under "blind" conditions in which everyone is injected in the same way but with a different substance, and neither the doctors nor the patients know who is receiving which substance.

According to Schorer, Arrowsmith is Lewis' best-plotted novel.[16] It was an instant success and, unlike some of his other works, caused no controversy. For his time, the subject was new, but he obviously understood the society well and apparently believed that it was changing for the worse. By today's standards the writing is somewhat simplistic, the satire too harsh, and many of the characters one-dimensional, but the story remains engrossing and instructive. In 1931 John Ford directed a movie version of *Arrowsmith* starring Ronald Coleman and Helen Hayes as Martin and Leora and featuring Myrna Loy as Joyce Lanyon. In 1999 a Czech film based on the novel appeared, proving the enduring appeal of Lewis' engaging work.

## REFERENCES

1 Lewis S (1925). *Arrowsmith*. New York: Signet Classic; 1961.
2 Schorer M. Afterword to *Arrowsmith*, by S Lewis. New York: Signet Classic; 1961. p. 431.

3 Lewis, op. cit., p. 433.

4 Lewis S. *Autobiography*. Available at: www.nobelprize.org/nobel_prizes/literature/laureates/1930/lewis-autobio.html

5 Ibid.

6 Wikipedia. *Sinclair Lewis*. Available at: http:/en.wikipedia.org/wiki/Sinclair_Lewis

7 Lewis, op. cit., *Arrowsmith*. p. 11.

8 Ibid., p. 96.

9 Ibid., p. 38.

10 Ibid., p. 150.

11 Ibid., p. 266.

12 Ibid., p. 295.

13 Ibid., p. 300.

14 Ibid., p. 426.

15 Ibid., p. 428.

16 Schorer, op. cit., p. 436.

**CHAPTER 5**

# Dr. Andrew Manson

## in *The Citadel*

### by A.J. Cronin[1]

---

### Themes

- Moral issues
- Combining practice with meaningful research
- Lung diseases related to coal mining
- Book's impact on society: might have influenced the birth of the National Health Service in Britain

---

Archibald Joseph (A.J.) Cronin (1896–1981) wrote *The Citadel* in 1937, barely two years before the outbreak of World War II, yet it belongs to a bygone era when the prevailing writer's mission was to draw the line between good and evil, between the noble and despicable. The novel, however, exposed the inequity and incompetence of the medical profession and made a big impact on the society of Great Britain.

Cronin was a physician whose accurate accounts of medical practice and problems prove that the book is largely autobiographical. Further evidence comes from his autobiography, *Adventures in Two Worlds*,[2] published in 1935. He graduated from the University of Glasgow Medical School in Scotland with highest honors, being awarded an M.B. and a Ch.B. He earned additional degrees, including a diploma in public health (1923) and his M.R.C.P. in 1924. In 1925, he was awarded a doctor degree (similar to an American Ph.D.) from the University of Glasgow for his dissertation, entitled *The History of Aneurysm*.[3] He practiced in the Scottish mining town of Tannochbrae and later in another mining town, Tredegar in South Wales. It was from Tredegar

41

that Cronin studied for advanced medical degrees, using books shipped to him from the Medical Library and riding a motorcycle to Cardiff to work in the pathology laboratory there. He was a naval surgeon during World War I and later became a medical inspector of mines, investigating occupational diseases in the coal industry. He married Agnes Mary Gibson, a doctor who apparently never practiced, with whom he had two children. Later he bought a practice in a rundown section of London and acquired more prosperous patients after he saved the life of an elderly wealthy woman living in a fashionable section of town abutting his own, who had swallowed liniment containing belladonna, mistaking it for her stomach medicine. She became his patient and sent to him other well-heeled friends. In his memoir, Cronin is unabashed in telling how he dealt with his rich, spoiled and neurotic patients. "I even invented a new disease for them – asthenia. This word, which means no more than weakness or general debility, became a sort of talisman . . ."[4] Naturally he also came up with a cure, a series of intramuscular injections that quickly became in vogue, as much the mode and as eagerly sought after as Manuel's new spring gowns. He admitted to having been a great rogue at this period but justified his behavior by saying:

> Asthenia gave these bored and idle women an interest in life. My tonics braced their languid nerves. I dieted them, insisted on a regime of moderate exercise and early hours. I even persuaded two errant wives to return to their long-suffering husbands, with the result that within nine months they had other matters than asthenia to occupy them.[5]

When Cronin developed a chronic duodenal ulcer, which his doctor assured him would perforate if he didn't take some time off to rest, he sold his practice, rented a place in Inveraray and wrote *Hatter's Castle*, the first of his long line of hugely successful novels. He never practiced medicine again. Another of his novels, *The Stars Look Down*, which examines social injustice in a north England mining community from 1903 to 1933, is considered by some a classic work of 20th-century British fiction. His novels deal with moral conflicts between the individual and society. His idealistic heroes expose corruption and seek justice for the downtrodden working class. Many of Cronin's books were best-sellers and were translated into numerous languages.[6]

## THE NOVEL

*The Citadel*'s hero, reminiscent of Martin Arrowsmith in the novel by Sinclair Lewis, is Dr. Andrew Manson. Manson is a member of the noble Scottish poor, son of a Highland woman and a Fifeshire farmer, orphaned at 18 with a schol-arship to study at St. Andrews University. He gets through medical school at Dundee with a loan of £250 from the Glen Endowment, set up by Sir Andrew Glen for worthy students with the given name of Andrew.[7] The need to pay back this money is what has brought Andrew to Wales, where the salaries for beginners are higher than are those for the job he really wanted – a clinical appointment at the Edinburgh Royal Hospital. Andrew's career can be fol-lowed as a voyage to five successive locations.

To begin with, he is just out of medical school when he arrives in Blaenelly, the township in an isolated Welsh mining valley, as an assistant to Dr. Page. When the novel opens, he is full of optimism, hope and excitement at finally starting his career but scared that his training isn't adequate and that he won't do well. His first discovery, no hint of which was part of his correspondence with the doctor's wife, is that Page suffered a stroke, is severely incapacitated and probably will not recover. The practice is controlled by Mrs. Page, a greedy woman who means to exploit Manson and appropriate for herself the money brought in by the practice. She misleads the Workers' Committee that controls healthcare in the town, insisting that Dr. Page will get well, playing on their loyalty to keep them from turning the practice over to Manson.

The mine is the only employer in town and each of the three doctors has his list of workers. The doctors' income is based on the number of patients they treat. Their assistants, like Manson, earn meager wages but accept these jobs because it is one way for a poverty-stricken young doctor to start in practice if he does not have the funds to go on to graduate study or to set up his own office. Assistants are medical slave laborers, obligated to respond to calls at any hour of the day or night, with no regular hours or time off.

Manson is an idealist with an impetuous and ardent nature. His first medi-cal challenge is a woman with fever that he is unable to diagnose, and he is feeling miserably inadequate until Dr. Denny, assistant to one of the other doctors and the cynical antidote to Manson's naive idealism, tells him that typhoid fever is endemic here because of a polluted well in one part of town and generally inadequate sewerage. Manson throws himself into attending to the five cases of typhoid that pop up after Denny explains that there is no use in calling the corrupt and lazy health officer, Dr. Griffiths, who won't come or do anything about the sanitation problem. Andrew isolates the sick, orders all water to be boiled, insists that a carbolic-soaked sheet cover each doorway, and disinfects latrines with pounds of chloride of lime. After a month all his patients improve and the practice starts growing as word travels through the mine that a good and caring doctor has come. Andrew overcomes his initial feelings of inadequacy when he makes a series of correct diagnoses while witnessing the incompetence of some of his older colleagues. He is slowly starting to understand that Denny may be right criticizing the state of English medicine, and that much of what he learned in medical school is not applicable to his practice, which means that he must start thinking for himself. He is flattered when Joe Morgan, a foreman driller at the mine, comes with his 43-year-old wife to announce a pregnancy after 20 barren years of marriage and tells Andrew they have delayed their plans to leave for South Africa, where he can earn more money in the gold mines, because they want him to deliver the baby. He even gets up enough nerve to join Denny in his plan to blow up the sewer, despite sincere scruples about breaking the law and fear of being caught and losing his career, which means everything to him. But they do it secretly and successfully and get a new sewer. His life brightens when he falls in love with the local schoolteacher, Christine Barlow.

Meanwhile he makes very astute diagnoses. An episode which made a big impression on one of the authors of this book (BS) when he read it while in medical school was the case of personality change of the workman Emrys, who unexpectedly became uncontrollably violent. Dr. Bramwell wants to commit him to the insane asylum; needing another doctor to co-sign the commitment papers, he calls on Andrew, who, from observing Emrys' skin and face, diagnoses thyroid deficiency resulting in a readily curable myxedema that had caused the psychosis. In the case of the unresponsive newborn Morgan baby, Andrew revives the infant by immersing him in alternate basins of hot and cold water and massaging the chest.

The romance with Chris proceeds. She accompanies him to a medical convention in Cardiff, where they visit exhibits advertising ineffective remedies and instructing doctors how to increase their incomes.

The Blaenelly episode comes to an end when Joe Morgan insists on giving Andrew five guineas as a thank you for saving his child. Andrew deposits the check in the bank in his own name and is accused by Blodwen Page of thievery, the bank manager having squealed. Andrew gives his notice and starts job hunting. There is an opening in Aberalaw, 30 miles away, a bigger town with more amenities and a real hospital. Andrew bests the other candidates and gets the job. He marries Chris and they go off to their new life.

At Aberalaw Andrew is at first thrilled; he envisions working at the hospital, saving lives and doing research. But slowly he finds a more subtle corruption than in simple Blaenelly. Dr. Llewellyn, the chief, who lives in a grand house and drives a handsome car, is a thoroughly competent physician and charmer, but he demands and pockets one-fifth of all the assistants' salaries. Llewellyn attends to all hospital cases because the assistants have no hospital privileges.

Andrew finds that most of the patients crowding his surgery are there to obtain disability certificates so they get paid for not working. When Andrew refuses one to a burly workman named Chenkin, he not only gains his eternal enmity but that of his whole family as well, and soon patients are asking to be transferred from his list to those of the other assistants. He also manages to antagonize the district nurse, who refuses to follow his orders. Andrew's fortunes improve when Owen, the respected secretary of the Committee, asks if he can be on Andrew's list.

Andrew observes again all that is wrong: the competition that drives the assistants apart and the unfairness of having them do all the initial work and leave the "cream" to Llewellyn. He tries to organize the other assistants to rebel against the cut of their salary taken by Llewellyn, but they won't stand together and he fails. Trying to figure out why this bugs him so much, Chris tells him he's just jealous, and not only of Llewellyn's excellence, but of his first-class qualifications. This sets Andrew off on a new tack, to study for the M.R.C.P., the most difficult of the hurdles to advancement, which requires the candidate to know two languages (Latin, French, German or Greek) before he can sit for the exam. Chris offers to teach him Latin and French. He acquires books from the London branch of the International Medical Library to study biochemistry and other subjects. He acquires a motorcycle and commutes to Cardiff to work in the pathology laboratory. During his orals he impresses the examiner with the knowledge that Paré was not the discoverer of aneurysm, because Celsus, a second-century Greek philosopher, had already mentioned aneurismus 13 centuries earlier.[7] With this kind of performance Andrew Manson gets his M.R.C.P.

Back at the mine there's a cave in. Manson descends with the miners to rescue Sam Bevan, whose arm is pinned under the fallen debris. He amputates it right there without anesthesia before the rest of the area collapses on them. His reputation is more significantly enhanced by this deed than by his degree, and his patients start returning.

But Andrew has more important things on his mind. As the result of many painstaking examinations he has become nearly certain that the large per-centage of the anthracite drillers who suffered from an insidious form of lung disease in Blaenelly, and who came to him complaining of a cough or a bit of phlegm in the tubes, were actually incipient or even open cases of pulmonary tuberculosis. Because he is finding the same thing here, "He began to ask himself if there was not some direct connection between the occupation and the disease."[8] He conceives a research project and obtains permission to do a systematic examination of all the workers in the three anthracite sinkings, using the pit workers and surfacemen as controls.

As Christmas approaches, life is very good for the Mansons: Chris is pregnant, Andrew's work is going well, they are well liked in the town. But by summer their luck has turned. Chris loses the baby when she falls through a rotting bridge on their property the Committee had delayed fixing and can't have more children. (Is it coincidence that Leora in Arrowsmith also loses her first baby and cannot have another?)

By 1927 Andrew finishes his research, which shows plain evidence of the marked preponderance of lung disease among the anthracite workers. Not only that, he has found the culprit – silica dust.[9] Using a dozen guinea pigs, he demonstrates that the dust causes abscesses when injected under the skin. He publishes the paper and also sends it off as a thesis to earn his doctorate at the university.

The roller-coaster rhythm of this novel – a downside to every triumph – continues. Chenkin will have his revenge. He manages to bring Manson before the committee set up to inquire about Andrew's vivisection and experiments on animals without a license. The hearing is stormy, full of meaningless accusations. "Why don't he give no medicine?", "Why was he wasting our time and money running off to Cardiff twice a week?", "Why don't he give proper certificates to the men?", "How could he turn Vale View into a slaughter house?"[10] Andrew defends himself.

> "Why do you men take white mice and canaries down the mine? To test for black damp – you all know that. And when the mice get finished by a whiff of gas – do you call that cruelty? No you don't. You realize that these animals have been used to save men's lives, perhaps your own lives. That's what I've been trying to do for you. I've been working on these lung diseases that you get from the dust in the mine headings. You all know that you get chest trouble and that when you do get it you don't get compensation. For these last three years I've spent nearly every minute of my spare time on this inhalation problem. I've found out something which might improve your working conditions, give you a fairer deal, keep you in health."[11]

Then he shows them the letter that awards him his M.D. for his work on dust inhalation. The committee of course decides in his favor. But Andrew has had it with Aberalaw and resigns. His paper, in the *Journal of Industrial Health in England*, and a brochure in the U.S. published by the Association of American Hygiene, do not make many waves, but one reaches Richard Stillman in Oregon, who compliments him and tells him that the active destructive ingredient in silicon is serecite. A letter arrives while he is vacationing in France, informing Andrew that the Coal Mines and Metalliferous Fatigue

Board has decided, because of his paper, to appoint a medical officer to look into the issue of silica and was offering him the job. Next stop, London.

The CMMF Board turns out to be a bureaucratic morass; no one works more than six hours a day; the Board takes forever to meet and assigns him meaningless projects before he can start on further dust research. Andrew realizes this is not for him and quits, thinking to buy a practice. Later he learns that Lord Ungar raised the matter of dust inhalation in the House of Commons, quoting freely from medical evidence given him by Dr. Maurice Gadsby, one of the MFB members. Gadsby was acclaimed by the Press as a Humanitarian and a Great Physician and silicosis was finally recognized as an industrial disease.[12]

Chris wants to move to the country, but Andrew has his heart set on staying in London. They find a practice they can afford in a run-down neighborhood. It's slow going at first but gradually patients come, mostly poor people who pay three and sixpence for their consultations. After a week Andrew begins to wonder if he'd made a horrible mistake in taking on this derelict practice. He thinks bitterly that, at age 30, he has his M.D. and M.R.C.P., he has clinical ability and a fine piece of clinical research work to his credit. Yet he's taking in barely enough three and sixpences to keep them in bread. He blames the system but still says, "I must succeed; damn it all, I will succeed."[13]

Andrew does succeed, beyond his wildest dreams. Miss Cramb, a saleswoman at the fancy clothing shop Laurier's, which borders the area of Andrew's practice, consults him about dermatitis on her hands that hasn't responded to any treatment recommended by the many doctors she's consulted. Manson diagnosis the cause as a blood condition and recommends a special diet, which cures the ever grateful Miss Cramb. She starts sending him rich patients. Little by little Andrew abandons his strict principles of proper medical practice. He gives needless allergy injections and takes kickbacks from the surgeon, Charles Ivory. He obtains a hospital appointment at Victoria Chest Hospital, buys new suits from a good tailor, purchases a car, takes an office in the fashionable West End, decides that he enjoys raking in money, doesn't always take Chris along to fashionable lunches, no longer has scruples about overprescribing or taking kickbacks, acquires a mistress and makes Chris' life completely miserable.

On one occasion, we meet up with Sir Dudley Rumbold-Blane, M.D. F.R.C.P., famous physician and member of the board of Cremo products. Rumbold's contributions to the health of the British public include excising a portion of the intestine on the grounds that it isn't needed (the Rumbold-Blane excision); introducing bran, yoghurt and the lactic acid bacillus into the British diet; writing menus for a famous restaurant chain; and pushing Cremogen as an enormously effective immune system strengthener which allows people to fight off the flu. One thing about Cronin: he may move papier mâché characters around the chessboard of his novels to make valid points about his contemporary society, but he certainly remains timely, even to this day.

Denny returns to London from years of wandering and gets a good surgical appointment but is not impressed by Andrew's success. When Andrew introduces Denny to Hope, a young biologist he met at the MFB, they both make fun of Manson and he is sharply defensive.

As she observes the changes in Manson, Chris is appalled but silent. Finally, she speaks up. "Oh! Don't you see, don't you see, you're falling a victim to the very system you used to run down, the thing you used to hate?"[14]

Andrew, wildly defensive at this attack, reminds her that people judge you by what you have, that have-nots get ordered about and that he intends to do the ordering in the future. "Now do you understand? Don't even mention this damned nonsense to me again."[15] Chris obeys but not before she tells him he'll be sorry.

And sorry Andrew surely is.

The truth of where he has arrived becomes clear only after he refers one of his poorer patients, the cobbler Vidler, to Ivory for the removal of a cyst. The surgeon, who has done only minor routine procedures for Andrew, is unable to handle this case because the cyst is hemorrhagic and, after opening it, he cannot stop the bleeding, allowing the patient to bleed to death. Andrew in his rage calls Ivory a butcher and the light dawns. He begs Chris' forgiveness and they enjoy a tender reconciliation. He decides to sell the practice, proposing to Hope and Denny that they form a group similar to what's being done in the U.S. and practice honest medicine together. But before this happens, Andrew suffers the loss of his wife and a threat to his license to practice medicine. Chris, now made joyful by Andrew's reversion into the man she knew and loved, rushes out to buy his favorite cheese for a late supper she's fixed and steps in front of a bus in her haste. She's dead on the spot.

In the meantime Stillman has come to London to set up a TB hospital similar to what he's done successfully in the States. Stillman's reputation is based not only on his highest technical skill but also on originality amounting almost to genius.

Mary, the daughter of an Aberalaw friend, has TB. Andrew admits her to the Victoria Hospital, where she undergoes an old-fashioned ineffective therapy. Andrew suggests performing a pneumothorax to her attending physician, who refuses. Manson tells Mary to sign herself out of Victoria, drives her to Stillman's sanatorium and stays to help Stillman with the procedure.

A coalition of two dishonest physicians offended by Manson and a disgruntled nurse lodge a complaint with the Licensing Council that Andrew collaborated with a foreigner who is not a physician. He is in danger of being struck from the registry.

Andrew's lawyer thinks that the only hope of saving his career is to show that Mary was Andrew's patient initially, that he had a personal interest in the case and naturally wanted to take it back into his own hands without causing his senior colleague distress. And that he went to Stillman because he was seeking a place where he could care for his patient, that Stillman was merely helping him and that he received no money for her care. He assures the Council that he did not intend an offense against the medical code nor had any awareness that his conduct could be construed as infamous. Mary testifies that the clinic was excellent and that she is cured.

Andrew prepares an additional defense. He points out to the board that Pasteur, Ehrlich, Haffjine (a plague fighter in India), and Metchnikoff (a famous Russian bacteriologist) were not doctors. He compares Stillman with them, saying Stillman has

> ". . . done more against tuberculosis than any man living in this country. He's out-side the profession. Yes! But there are plenty inside it who have been running up against TB all their lives and have never done an atom of good in fighting it."[16]

On fire, Andrew cannot stop.

> "If we go on trying to make out that everything's wrong outside the profession and everything is right within, it means the death of scientific progress. We'll just turn into a tight little trade protection society. It's high time we started put-ting our own house in order . . . think of the hopelessly inadequate training doctors get. When I qualified I was more of a menace to society than anything else . . . Anything I know I've learned since then. But how many doctors do learn anything beyond the ordinary rudiments they pick up in practice? They haven't got the time, poor devils; they're rushed off their feet. That's where our whole organization is rotten. We ought to be arranged in scientific units. There ought to be compulsory post-graduate classes. There ought to be a great attempt to bring science to the front line . . . give every practitioner a chance to study, to co-operate in research. And what about commercialism? The useless guinea-chasing treatments, the unnecessary operations, the crowds of worthless pseudo-scientific proprietary preparations we use – isn't it time some of these were eliminated? The whole profession is too intolerant and smug."[17]

The Council sides with Andrew after this brave speech and he is free to start a new chapter in his professional life in partnership with Denny and Hope.

In judging this immensely popular book by current literary standards, the writing is somewhat simplistic, clichés abound and the characters are either good or bad with not much in between. The improbable changes Manson undergoes in his voyage from idealism to greed and back are somewhat incredible. And where in the real world are women like Christine? Pure, honest, charming, intelligent, erudite, idealistic, dedicated, supportive, tender, generous, unselfish, feminine and tactful, with wonderful taste and intuition? And a good cook!

In his upbeat and heroic moments Andrew Manson is impressive – the amputation at the mine, which Cronin actually did in his brief career, the diagnosis of myxedema psychosis, and the difficult delivery and revival of the stillborn baby. However, in his series of conflicts with his peers and authority figures, Manson comes across as idealistic but self-righteous, conceited, uncompromising, stubborn and completely unable to disguise his contempt for incompetence, laziness and corruption.

Cronin does a fine job of highlighting the faults of the system – the paucity of clinical research, the environmental devastation caused by coal mining, the ignorance of country doctors, the lack of post-graduate education, hospitals without X-rays and other essential equipment, a stifling bureaucracy at the CMMF Board, doctors' busy schedules including evening house calls, corruption in private practice, fee splitting, unnecessary follow-up appointments, difficulty of obtaining hospital privileges, prescribing many drugs though only a few were useful at the time, anti-vivisectionists hampering research. It seems that having earned the titles M.D. and M.R.C.P. does not matter as much as being affable, having the proper connections and willingly acceding to patients' demands, such as ear piercing. He also catalogs the attributes of a good researcher: careful review of the existing knowledge, formulation of hypotheses, testing them in animal models and clinical experiments. And the qualities of a good practitioner: thorough, honest, using few drugs, but, if the drug is effective, such as potassium bromide in epilepsy, using it in doses that make possible the assessment of its effectiveness.

Naturally they made a movie of *The Citadel* (in 1938), directed by King Vidor, with Robert Donat playing Andrew Manson, Rosalind Russell (an unlikely choice because of her Hollywood sophistication) as perfect and patient Christine, and Ralph Richardson as Denny.

Peter E. Dans, M.D., reviewing the movie in the fall 1994 issue of *The Pharos*, calls the movie old-fashioned but says it has a soul. He points out that the book is much more critical of doctors' ethical lapses than the movie is, and that it received scathing criticism in *JAMA* for painting "not a fair picture of medicine in either Great Britain or the United States." On the other hand, he quotes Dr. High Cabot of the Mayo Clinic writing to the American publishers as follows:

> The book appears to be so important that I should be glad to believe that it would be at the disposal of every medical student and practitioner under 35 in this country. . . . I can say at once that there is no important situation which he draws, the counterpart of which cannot be found in this country.[18]

*The Citadel* may be the only book in our series that had profoundly practical effects. It has been rumored that this book played a major role not only in the battle to establish the National Health Service in England in 1948, but also in the election of the Labour Government in 1945 that made the NHS a reality.[19,20] It therefore stands, with all its faults, as a tribute to the transforming power of literature. The medical aid scheme found in Tredegar, where the miners paid a small weekly contribution to a special fund and were entitled to free medical care, became the basis for the form of socialized medicine adopted in Britain after World War II, the credit going to Aneurin Bevan, Minister of Health, who had been a miner in Tredegar.

## REFERENCES

1 Cronin AJ (1937). *The Citadel*. Boston, New York, London: Little, Brown and Company; 1965.
2 Cronin AJ (1935). *Adventures in Two Worlds*. Chicago: Peoples Book Club; 1952.
3 Ibid., p. 168.
4 Ibid., p. 196.
5 Ibid., p. 197.
6 Wikipedia. *A. J. Cronin*. Available at: http://en.wikipedia.org/wiki/A._J._Cronin
7 Cronin, op. cit., *The Citadel*. p. 14.
8 Ibid., p. 172.
9 Ibid., p. 178.
10 Ibid., p. 184.
11 Ibid., pp. 184–5.
12 Ibid., p. 210.
13 Ibid., p. 216.
14 Ibid., p. 277.
15 Ibid., p. 278.
16 Ibid., p. 363.
17 Ibid., p. 364.
18 Dans PE. The Citadel. *Pharos*. 1994; **57**(4): 36–7.
19 Samuels R. North and South. *London Review of Books*. 1995; **17**(12): 3–6.
20 Harrison C, Gough PB. Conversations: compellingness in reading research. *Reading Res Q*. 1986; **31**(3): 334–41.

# CHAPTER 6

# Dr. Lucas Marsh

## in *Not as a Stranger*

### by Morton Thompson[1]

---

### Themes

- A doctor obsessed with medicine, who sees nothing beyond it
- The broad range of activities of a general practitioner before specialization in medicine
- The County Medical Society, which protects the physician's image and does not expose the "rotten apples"
- Hurried doctor lacks time for a thorough work-up of patients

---

Before creating *Not as a Stranger*, Morton Thompson (1908–53) wrote *The Cry and the Covenant*, a novel describing the life of the Viennese physician Ignaz Semmelweiss, who had deduced that the unwashed hands of operators in the delivery room were responsible for the high mortality of newborns and their mothers from sepsis known as puerperal fever. It is believed that Thompson's interest in medicine came from his unfulfilled desire to become a physician, and it is possible that the obsession with medicine of Lucas March, the hero of this novel, reflects the author's own passion for medical life. It is unknown how long Thompson labored on this vast sprawling medical panorama in a book whose name derives from a passage in the Book of Job. Appearing post-humously in 1954, the nearly 1000-page narrative tells the story of Luke Marsh from boyhood through college, medical school and the early years of medical practice in a small town in an unspecified American state. The action takes place in the early 20th century, ending in the midst of the ruinous depression of the late thirties, before World War II. This book, which sold a million and a half copies and topped the list of best-selling novels in the year it was issued, is still read today, possibly because the problems of the doctor–patient relationship, the moral challenges of the profession and the role of the physician in an era of phenomenal progress in the more effective and broadened scope of medical practice are still pertinent today. Despite the sentimental, unpolished and unsophisticated writing (when it is judged by modern standards), the novel remains rewarding and heartwarming for the contemporary physician and layperson. The narrative moves smoothly, captivating the reader's interest with dramatic action, skillful storytelling and vivid dialogues, even though the characters are largely one-dimensional and predictably evoke sympathy or antipathy as their standards of integrity and morality become apparent from the description of their physical features, facial expressions, attire, language and mannerisms.

## THE NOVEL

Luke's obsession with medicine begins early in childhood as he accompanies the local physician on house calls in a horse-drawn buggy and when he is allowed to explore the instruments and browse through the medical texts in the doctor's office. His home situation is dismal, with a constant feud between his overprotective, neurotic and mystical mother and his crude, poorly educated, philandering father, who is bent on continuing the expansion of his horse harness business, oblivious to the growing production of automobiles that will inevitably end horse-drawn transportation. Neither of the parents is sympathetic to his dreams of becoming a doctor, but his early studies proceed unimpeded. He sustains himself in college by a variety of menial jobs and by depriving himself of anything beyond bare subsistence, but his drive toward a medical degree is stopped by "the pitiless eyes"[2] of the bursar, who denies him admission to medical school if he cannot pay the tuition. A part-time job is no longer an option, as medical school requires full-time attendance of lectures, followed by a succession of assignments to memorize volumes of information destined to be promptly forgotten. The inheritance left him by his mother, who dies early of throat cancer, was stolen by his father after he forged Luke's signature. The sources of borrowed money were exhausted. Undeterred, Luke conceives the idea of marrying someone with money. He casts his eye on Kristina, a head surgical nurse earning a good salary and saving much of it because her needs are modest. She is slightly older than he is but Luke doesn't hesitate to pounce on her fortune. Pretending to be madly in love, he courts this simple, decent and naive maiden of Swedish extraction from Minnesota until she accepts his marriage proposal. This gives him access to her savings, which he uses to complete medical school, internship and post-graduate medical and surgical residencies.

During his training Luke briefly explores an academic career but is quickly dissuaded from this path by his friend and classmate, Avery, who tells him that among the students only a handful of fellows genuinely like or love medicine, and once in a great while somebody appears who cannot imagine anything else, but that most of the students are tradesmen or are there because this is what their parents want them to do. Worse are the contingents of nuggeteers and prize-drunkards, and in every class, there is somebody who will become a menace to society. Among fellow teachers there will be some pompous asses on the platform proposing something that is obsolete or downright false.

Finally, Luke becomes a practitioner. The seemingly insurmountable obstacles have been overcome, the dream has become reality and "The child who knew no other hope, whose world had no other meaning, stood now, fulfilled, on the threshold of Heaven."[3]

Ahead is the town of Greenville, where Luke is warmly received by the elderly Dr. Runkelman as a partner in his thriving surgical and medical practice, built up over 30 years. As a result of a one-night stand and an unfortunate prank played on him by his inebriated friends, Dr. Runkelman acquired syphilis as a young man. When Luke arrives in town, the syphilis has progressed to an enlarging aneurysm of the ascending aorta with aortic insufficiency. The diagnosis becomes obvious to Luke as he observes the doctor's chest motions, even though the description of the physical findings in this case is inaccurate – a rare lapse in the otherwise properly coached use of medical terminology throughout the text. (The author was indebted to Dr. Robert T. Morris, author of *Fifty Years as a Surgeon*.)

Dr. Runkelman is an experienced diagnostician and a skillful surgeon. After a morning filled with several operations, he sees up to 60 patients in his office in the afternoon, each paying him 75 cents or a dollar, a fee unchanged since he first came to town. This symptom-oriented practice leaves no time for comprehensive evaluation or for focusing on more complicated cases. Luke realizes that for a large number of patients the complaints are psychosomatic; the illnesses are imaginary and the drugs are no more than placebos. Luke is critical of the way Dr. Runkelman chooses not to turn anyone away, seeing them all but having little time for each one and risking mistakes, acknowledging that some may die unnecessarily because of incorrect diagnosis, and that some will do well against all expectation, and that this will not make any difference since "they will keep right on coming."[4] Luke vows that this will never be his problem. He accepts only one right way, which is a thorough examination of patients with real illnesses and refusing to deal with psychosomatic or imaginary complaints. He vows to be alone in his own practice of medicine in the office, hospital and laboratory.

Luke is very fond of Dr. Runkelman and two other physicians in town whom he respects. But he also observes doctors who are mere merchants, incompetent physicians harming their patients, and he sees a consultant stealing money from his wallet left in the pocket of his laboratory coat, presumably to compensate for a low consulting fee. He also becomes aware of doctors taking kickbacks from pharmacists, which raises the cost of drugs. At that time organized medicine lacked the means to protect the public from quacks, charlatans and ineffective or noxious remedies.

A different type of attack on the medical profession is launched by an iconoclastic lawyer, Ben Cosgrove, a shrill populist and self-proclaimed communist who accuses physicians of fostering the delusion of omniscience while trading on human ignorance and building a big business. He raves about doctors sometimes being scientists and, at other times, artists. He asserts, "You have never made up your mind which front you want to offer for your public's respect. You have got the will to obscure."[5] Luke does not argue with him.

In his practice Luke has to deal with end-of-life situations, which brings him into conflict with the existing practices that speed up the inevitable death by benign neglect or an overdose of narcotics. He is not overtly religious but endorses the sanctity of life to the last breath. In that era, modern long-term life-sustaining procedures were not yet available and most of Luke's heroic attempts to sustain a fading life are futile, but he clings to his conviction that "nobody is a goner"[6], even when the illness is terminal and incurable.

One of Luke's most despicable colleagues is Dr. Snider, the old, tobacco-stained, saliva-drooling director of the county hospital for the indigenous population, whom Dr. Runkelman calls a fool. This man is so careless giving ether anesthesia that Runkelman prefers to avoid ether, favoring spinal anesthesia instead. Dr. Snider sends incurable patients to unheated rooms in winter to accelerate their death by pneumonia and purposefully fails to tie bleeding arteries during a laparotomy after discovering an incurable disseminated malignancy. These are not the only acts of callousness and neglect of duty that inflame Luke's contempt for the old man, whose disastrous ignorance and incompetence Luke believes endanger patients' lives during surgery. One such episode of particularly bad judgment, a surgical procedure during which Dr. Snider perforates the bowel, causing a hemorrhage that leads to the patient's death, is so upsetting to Luke that he takes the unusual step of denouncing Dr. Snider to the Medical Licensing Board and asking them to revoke his medical license. Not only is Luke's request flatly turned down, but also he is severely admonished by the chairman of the County

Medical Society that such action would be unacceptable. Having an M.D. diploma makes Dr. Snider "one of us", which, he tells Luke, is a part of you and a part of me to be protected by the Society regardless of how one practices medicine. "We are liable to errors in judgment, Doctor, all of us,"[7] he says, and therefore organized medicine must be protected. The public has a right to have faith in the medical profession. Therefore it is the duty of the medical profession to keep this faith whole. The chairman's final words are: "I refuse to entertain your charges. We are all doctors, and we are all in this together."[8] He warns Luke that, by pursuing these charges, he may become ostracized and subsequently defenseless against ever making a mistake.

In dramatizing this encounter, the author makes it very clear that the medical profession will not take action against incompetent and unscrupulous practitioners. The book ends before Dr. Marsh has an opportunity to make a serious error of judgment, but in the movie version of 1955, with Robert Mitchum as Dr. Marsh and Olivia de Havilland as Kristina, the story changes to the extent that Luke is forced to face his own morality after his misjudgment leads to the death of a friend.

Dr. Runkelman notices signs of fatigue in Luke and tries to tell him not to work so hard and not to take it all so seriously, but it is difficult to change him because Luke has no interests beyond medicine. This is the negative side of such professional addiction, threatening to produce a boring, uninformed, culturally deprived, asocial individual. This is made worse by the fact that sub-specialization was in its infancy and that most physicians were general practitioners, combining adult and pediatric medicine with surgery, which consisted mainly of appendectomy, tonsilectomy, cholecystectomy, relief of intestinal obstruction, herniorraphy and obstetrical care. Most of the remedies that were available before World War II have been abandoned during the second half of the 20th century.

As time goes on Kristina begins to embarrass Luke by her simple-mindedness, her annoying Swedish speech intonation when she calls him Lukey, and her lack of cultural refinement. He confesses to his friend that he does not love her, while she, unaware of his inner feelings, idealizes him in trustful adoration. Luke does not see what is obvious to his colleagues, who tell him how lucky he should feel having such a pleasant, good-looking companion who happens to be an exceptionally skillful and experienced nurse in the operating room.

When Kristina travels to stay with her dying father, Luke, left alone, begins to pursue Henrietta Lane, whom he had encountered at the meeting of the committee investigating the spread of infectious diseases through the water supply. She is a New Englander and graduated from an art school in New

York, but she has become resigned to the fact that she is not going to be a top-notch painter. She bemoans the necessity of making a living by decorating mass-produced cheap pottery and has no friends at her intellectual or artistic level. Observing the handsome Luke passionately involved in the discussion during the meeting, she makes note of his dull Swedish wife and guesses that there is nothing between them. She begins flirting with Luke. Their attraction is mutual and she becomes his lover, losing her virginity. The clandestine affair continues after pregnant Kristina returns home. Rumors of the affair reach Kristina, who becomes despondent and attempts to abort her pregnancy. She is thwarted by another physician, who appears accidentally on the scene just in time to persuade Kristina to vomit the pills she has taken. As an observant physician, Luke becomes aware of the changes in Kristina's physique, including enlarged nipples, but does not realize that she is three months pregnant. Until now Luke had firmly rejected the idea of having a family and was prepared to continue his liaison with his lover. But Henrietta puts an end to the affair by leaving town after losing her job – a victim of the economic depression.

At the end of the book Luke is persuaded to take part in a camping and hunting expedition, where he becomes lost in the woods. Fearing that he will perish alone, he becomes aware of the need for company, support and love. After he is rescued, he makes passionate love to his wife in a fairly explicit passage for 1954 and discovers in the process her pregnancy. Joyfully, he reconciles himself to becoming a father.

Reminiscing about his ruthless, deliberate deed of marrying an unloved woman to make it possible to become a physician, it finally dawns on him that his wife's integrity, devotion and exquisite skill as a nurse will make her an outstanding supporting partner in his medical practice. This happy ending is like a Hollywood movie, but the reader absorbed in the tale of Luke Marsh from his childhood to this point in time is tempted to wonder what lies ahead for our hero and his wife after their first child is born. Will Luke be an attentive father? Will Kristina, now a mother, have time to assist him in his practice? Will they plan a larger family? Will he be drafted into the service during World War II? Will he be able to continue to practice general medicine and surgery simultaneously without additional training and Board certification? Will he be drawn into medical politics? Will he temper his intolerance toward less scrupulous colleagues and become more forgiving? Will he have an active social life? Will he remain faithful to his wife?

And, for Kristina, will her adoration of Luke remain unbroken? Will she be able to keep his interest in her as his practice grows and elevates his stature in the community? Or will she share the fate of the many wives alienated and divorced when they are no longer useful, after having put their husbands through medical school and post-graduate training?

Finally, do we know people like them and like the other doctors in the book? If the answer is yes, the book is worth recommending to today's medical students and practitioners, so that they may compare the contemporary medical field with one of the recent past. The book also captures the devastating effects of the economic depression and the ravages of a typhoid epidemic caused by contaminated drinking water, and it even touches on anti-Semitism by exposing quotas for Jews seeking entrance to medical school and the blocking of a Jewish pathologist, Dr. Ahrens, from teaching and doing research there.

## REFERENCES

1 Thompson M (1935). *Not as a Stranger*. Bergenfield, N.J.: Signet Book from New American Library; 1954.
2 Ibid., p. 136.
3 Ibid., p. 356.
4 Ibid., p. 460.
5 Ibid., p. 487.
6 Ibid., p. 428.
7 Ibid., p. 733.
8 Ibid., p. 738.

# CHAPTER 7

# *Cancer Ward*

## by Aleksandr Solzhenitsyn[1]

---

### Themes

- Cancer hospital in an Asian Soviet Republic – drabness and crowding
- Stalin is dead, but his cult and oppressive policies persist
- High prevalence of women physicians
- Medical personnel lack protection from X-ray radiation
- Irrational expectations of cancer cure by an untested plant extract

---

## ALEKSANDR SOLZHENITSYN

The oppressive political terror pervading the Soviet Union, isolated from the rest of the world by an "iron curtain," was particularly hard on artists and writers required to conform in their works to the style and spirit of "social realism." Any deviation from the prescribed form, or an unorthodox look at the society, was punished by confiscation and destruction of the work, expulsion from the Professional Union, or worse. In this atmosphere, condemned either to silence or blatant insincerity, were some of the most talented Russian artists of the 20th century, including the writers Michael Bulgakov, Boris Pasternak, Vera Ginsburg and Vassily Grossman, the poet Ossip Mandelstam, the composer Dmitri Shostakovich and the cellist Mstislav Rostropovich. But in the annals of future history two giant figures, the physicist Andrei Sakharov and the novelist-historian Aleksandr Solzhenitsyn will be hailed for their moral vision and unflinching courage to face oppression.

Aleksandr Solzhenitsyn descended from an intellectual Cossack family. He was born in 1918 in Kislovodsk, a spa town in the Northern Caucasus. His father, an officer in the Tsarist army, died before Aleksandr's birth, and his mother supported herself and her son by working as a typist in Rostov, the city where

Solzhenitsyn attended university, studying mathematics and physics, with concomitant correspondence courses in literature from Moscow University. After his graduation in 1941, he was drafted into the army during World War II, advancing to the rank of captain of artillery. Although twice decorated and wounded in action, he was arrested in 1945 for criticizing Stalin – the man with the mustache – in an intercepted letter to a friend. He was sentenced to eight years in prison, to be followed by permanent exile. The knowledge of mathematics and physics helped him avoid hard labor much of the time and thus to survive prison and the camps. Between 1953 and 1956 Solzhenitsyn lived in exile in the village Kok-Terek in Kazakhstan. He supported himself as a teacher and also wrote in secret. After rehabilitation in 1957, he settled in Riazan as a teacher and wrote much but published little. His first major work, *One Day in the Life of Ivan Denisovich*, appeared in 1962 and marked the beginning of Soviet prison camp (gulag) literature. It was compared to Dostoyevsky's novel *House of the Dead*, but this account was more chilling because the victim in the story was not a criminal but an innocent naval officer. The next major work, *The First Circle* (1968), was also set in the system of prisons and concentration camps but was confiscated by the KGB. The same fate awaited his most famous work, *The Gulag Archipelago* (1973).

As with Pasternak, the Soviet Government denounced the Nobel Prize awarded to Solzhenitsyn in 1970, and the author was exiled from the Soviet Union in 1974. He moved to the United States in 1976, settling in Cavendish, Vermont, and focused his writing on the history of events that led to the Russian Revolution (in August 1914). After the collapse of the Soviet Union, he returned to Russia in 1994 as a devoted Russian Orthodox Christian and turned his critical pen to attacking Western materialism, but he has not spared current Russia's materialism within the business circles and government in Putin's Russia (*Russia Collapsing*, 1998). Solzhenitsyn died from a heart condition on August 3, 2008.

### Solzhenitsyn's cancer – a medical mystery

In his autobiography prepared for the Nobel Foundation in 1970, Solzhenitsyn claims to have developed a tumor while still in the camps in 1952, possibly skin cancer, according to one of his biographers, and he was operated on but apparently not cured, since at the end of 1953, while in exile in a village in Kazakhstan, his cancer progressed rapidly. He was unable to eat or sleep and was "near death, severely affected by poisons from the tumor."[2] The condition was cured in 1954 at a cancer clinic in Tashkent. Solzhenitsyn believes that the nature of his "tumor" was established later, presumably from a biopsy specimen, but how he was cured is not revealed. Judging from his own description of the available cancer therapy in this hospital, as described in his semi-autobiographical novel, *Cancer Ward*, it would have to have been a radiosensitive neoplasm.

## *CANCER WARD*

The novel was written in the 1960s, barred from publication in the Soviet Union, smuggled out of the country and published abroad. It is a passionate condemnation of the Stalinist regime viewed from the setting of a massive stone structure, erected in Tashkent 70 years ago and at that time housing a hospital for cancer victims. The action takes place when the author was hospitalized there in 1955, two years after Stalin's death. He delegates the role of narrator to his fictional alter ego, Oleg Kostoglotov, a man of similar age and with a similar life story (army, prison, camps, exile and cancer) and similar intelligence and powers of observation. One can imagine watching him as he stealthily tiptoes through the building, storing in his memory the pictures of different places and of people and their conversations. His curiosity takes him to the waiting room, with its mud-covered floor, and to corridors crowded with newly arrived patients awaiting a vacant hospital bed. He views wards with rows of between nine and 30 patient beds separated from each other only by a night table with a single drawer, the nurse's stations, the treatment rooms and the X-ray facilities. Having smuggled in and hidden under his bed his own boots, Oleg can leave the building and explore the outdoors.

He observes that most of the patients are native Uzbeks (Tashkent is a university town and capital of the Soviet Uzbek Republic), but there is a large contingent from the vast neighboring Kazakhstan, where the native Kazakhs have witnessed an influx of people from the region of Volga, which harbored centuries-old German settler communities, Chechens expelled from Caucasus, and Tatars from Crimea, entire nations uprooted by Stalin during the war and exiled to the inhospitable steppes and deserts of central Asia. There are also exiled Greeks and Kurds and prisoners serving their sentences in the wretched camps, condemned to permanent exile if they survived the terms of their prison sentences. The narrator observes their bodies deformed by malignant tumors and listens to their conversations. From the nuances and inflections of their speech he can recognize a criminal, a prison guard and a high official in the camp administration. From the family name of a young woman doctor he deduces her German extraction. In a heavy-set silent man sitting on the bench, who happens to be the exiled former professor Shulubin, he recognizes a man of kindred intelligence with whom he can talk about the system that thrives on false denunciations, mass arrests and deportations of innocent people, cruel judges in the service of the prosecution, extorted confessions of alleged anti-government plotting, and humiliation of political prisoners preyed upon by the criminal convicts.

From a slang expression used by the chief surgeon, he guesses correctly that his presence here is not purely voluntary, and when he peers into a book read by a tired cleaning woman after work, he recognizes the French text revealing an educated person and he can envision the thorny road leading to her present existence. From a pert medical student who works as a nurse, he borrows a textbook of pathological anatomy to understand the different forms of neoplasms. He is passionate and angry when encountering injustice and is full of sarcasm and contempt during political debates with patients defending the regime.

Unlike the author, Kostoglotov is not cured when discharged from the hospital to return to the village where he worked as a mechanic. He will mourn his dog, shot in his absence by a drunkard, he may marry another exile in the village before he dies, and he will remember the apricot tree in full bloom, spotted in the yard of a house in Tashkent's old quarter.

## DOCTORS AND MEDICAL TREATMENT

Narrating this subject, the author was on a less firm ground. His knowledge of medical procedures and drugs was limited, and it is not likely that his status as an exiled political prisoner would provide him access to the private lives and living quarters of physicians or nurses portrayed in the book. Thus it is no longer an account of a witness but a product of the author's imagination. Nevertheless, it is probably a truthful assessment.

Of the 10 physicians at the hospital, there are three men and seven women. One of the men is the medical director, bearing a title of a senior doctor. He is named Nizamatadin Bahramowicz and is an Uzbek born in a mountain village. As a privileged native and a shrewd conformist, he climbed to this position of nearly unlimited power, allowing him to appoint and promote favorite employees lacking qualifications for the job – a sort of affirmative action for advancing the local population. One of them is a young Uzbek doctor assigned to the operating room even though he cannot operate. The senior doctor's ward rounds serve two purposes: to search the contents of the patients' night tables for prohibited items and to urge the discharge of those who were doomed or not likely to improve. Their discharge before death boosted the hospital census of less sick patients and lowered the mortality rates.

Lev Leonidovich is one of the two competent surgeons. The other is an experienced chain-smoking woman, Yevgenia Ustinova. The busy operative schedule has been designed for five surgeons, but since the young Uzbek and two young women appointed by the senior doctor are totally useless in the operating room, the schedule has to be fulfilled by the two capable but constantly overloaded doctors.

The four radiologists, performing both the diagnostic examinations and X-ray therapy, are women who also handle blood transfusions. The X-ray tubes apparently lack proper shielding, and there is no mention that the personnel carried dosimeters to check their radiation exposure. The senior woman, Ludmila Afanasyevna Dontsova, who has been exposed to this environment for 20 years, suffers from radiation sickness, and her white blood cell count is only 2000 when the story is told. In describing one afternoon in her life, readers can appreciate how poorly the physicians are paid. This 50-year-old experienced department head, a respected author of several scientific communications, wears an old ill-fitting dress, travels home in a rickety trolley and stands in a long line in a government store to receive, with an apparent joy, a precious bottle of sunflower oil and a kilogram of minced ham sausage. She arrives at her modest apartment to do the family wash and cook dinner because her husband and son, like most Russian men, do not help with domestic chores. Dr. Dontsova is very tired, but her fatigue is not caused solely by overwork. She has suspected for some time that there is a malignant growth in her digestive tract, and when the examination with barium swallow (there is no mention of endoscopy) confirms her suspicion, she is sent to Moscow for treatment.

Of her junior staff, attention is focused on 35-year-old Vera Kornilyevna Gangart, who had lost her fiancé 14 years before, during World War II, and has been alone since the completion of her medical studies. This is the fate of many women because the war casualties created a huge imbalance between the male and female population. At least she has her own room in a communal apartment. One evening she stares at the photograph of her young fiancé, really still a boy, and compares her love to an agave plant that blooms only once in its lifetime.

Vera transfuses blood to Oleg Kostoglotov, and although his diagnosis is not revealed, she admonishes him to submit to the prescribed intravenous injections of sinestrol (an estrogen preparation), which for us is an incomprehensible choice of therapy. Oleg, however, is reluctant to receive estrogen, not for this reason, but because of his fear of becoming impotent.

Another strange medication is colloidal gold, which is impatiently awaited by a young geologist entering the cancer ward with malignant melanoma and probably metastases. He hopes to be cured by this medication if it can somehow be procured by his mother, a doctor in Moscow. The standard therapy includes glucose infusions and a drug, ambigene, but there is no evidence of chemotherapy, since the mainstays of treatment are radical surgery and radiation.

The patients are stirred by the widely circulating rumor about the discovery of a cancer cure in an extract from a fungus named chaga growing on birch trees. A researcher, Maslennikov, had observed that the peasants in his district brewed chaga as a substitute for real tea and had no cancer, connecting the two observations in his mind. But even in the absence of proof that chaga cures cancer for all patients with advanced malignancy, this treatment becomes a ray of hope to which the patients cling while awaiting scientific confirmation and the release of the alternative treatment. This is similar to the hopes of cancer patients in the United States expecting to be cured by laetrile, who remained undeterred by publications reporting the complete ineffectiveness of this compound.

Even after Stalin's death, the Soviet doctors live in fear of denunciation for alleged errors in practice, particularly when caring for political bigwigs. An illustrative episode is recounted by Lev Leonidovich, who was summoned to serve on a type of grand jury called to judge a surgeon. The surgeon was required to explain his actions during an operation that resulted in the death of a child with intestinal volvulus. The grand jury members included some laypersons and some professional experts. The purpose of the proceedings was to determine whether the case should be tried in a regular court. Lev Leonidovich recounts how his passionate speech in defense of the accused colleague contributed to his acquittal, with only a rebuke for incomplete record keeping. He says that the accused was lucky to be a Russian, because the verdict might have been different if he was a German or a "y-yid" (kike). He expresses his opposition to the trial of physicians by laypeople but is reminded by Dr. Ustinova that sometimes public prosecution may be appropriate, citing cases of swabs left in the stomach, saline injected instead of novocaine, transfusion with the wrong blood type or the development of gangrene of the leg within an improperly applied cast. Their discussion continues, but procedural changes are hardly expected, as can be deduced from the closing remarks made by the chief city-surgeon: "Comrades, putting doctors on trial shows superb initiative, truly superb."[3]

Reflecting on Solzhenitsyn's account of conditions on the Cancer Ward, it appears to be mainly of historical interest, but the suffering of cancer patients and their families remains universal. As long as the cure of these diseases evades us and the lives of children or adults in the prime of life cannot be saved, the physician in charge of such patients must gain understanding of how to deal with their fears, denials and false hopes in the most humane manner.

It is not difficult to understand Solzhenitsyn's bitterness after all his suffering imposed by the Soviet regime, but some gratitude would be in order for curing his cancer. One can also speculate that he owes his cure, in part, to a system of free universal health care in which a convict and a high party dignitary share the same multi-bed hospital ward and undergo the same treatment. But his vision for the future Russia is a country without political prisoners and without omnipotent party dignitaries.

## REFERENCES

1 Solzhenitsyn A (1968). *The Cancer Ward*. Translated from the Russian by N Bethell and D Burg. New York: Farrar, Straus & Giroux; 1969.
2 Bjorkegren H. *Alexander Solzhenitsyn: a biography*. New York: Third Press; 1972.
3 Solzhenitsyn, op. cit., p. 370.

# CHAPTER 8

# Doctors on the island of Capri

## *The Story of San Michele*
by Dr. Axel Munthe[1]

## *An Impossible Woman: The Memoirs of Dottoressa Moor*
by Elisabeth Moor with an introduction by Graham Greene[2]

---

### Themes

- Society doctor who also treats the poor free of charge
- Doctor as art lover and collector
- Psychosomatic medicine and hypnosis
- Male chauvinist doctor
- Woman doctor practicing ethical medicine with selfless courage while reminiscing about her lovers

---

When one of us (BS) was in medical school in the 1930s, a best-seller translated into a multitude of languages, including one he spoke at that time, introduced him to the autobiography of the Swedish physician Axel Munthe, *The Story of San Michele*. This book sank into some crevasse of his treasured reminiscences and he was pleasantly surprised when, 60 years later, a salesman at the Borders bookstore in Indianapolis told him that copies of this book could be ordered. The paperback edition arrived, its cover picturing the sculptures and marble columns adorning the portico of Axel Munthe's Villa San Michele in Anacapri, on the island of Capri in the Bay of Naples. The book first appeared in the United States in 1929. By 1930, there had been 12 editions of the English version alone.[3] The copyright was removed in 1957, and the memoir that arrived was a second printing from 1991. It received outstanding reviews for its imaginative style.

The adolescent Munthe spent little time in his native Sweden, instead practicing medicine primarily in Paris and Italy. He was the youngest M.D. ever graduated in France. A handsome polyglot, he became the favorite physician of foreign residents and visitors in the two capitals, attracting the rich, the famous, the aristocrats, the artists and the writers, plus many neurotic women. Although professing indifference to monetary rewards, he must have earned sufficient sums to be able to purchase land on the site of the ruins of the villa of the Roman emperor Tiberius on the island of Capri, to build a castle-like home there and to acquire a collection of exquisite art from antiquity and the Renaissance.

Non-surgical medicine at the end of 19th century dealt mainly with infections and, before the emergence of antibiotics, Axel Munthe could have had little impact on the course of epidemics of typhoid fever, cholera and scarlet fever, nor could he have prevented the ravages of diphtheria among the non-vaccinated population, since the vaccine developed by Behring became available only in 1892. Thus the clue to his proclaimed therapeutic triumphs must have been his understanding of psychosomatic illness and the maladies of imagination. These conditions were often curable, which enhanced his reputation, spreading an aura of fame and adulation. While in Paris, Munthe was a pupil of Charcot, the idolized neurologist who, following the practices of Franz Mesmer (1734–1815), presided each Tuesday over dramatic séances at the Salpêtrière Hospital, gathering physicians, artists, actors, writers and fashionable demimondes, to whom he demonstrated the power of hypnosis, usually on selected hysterical women patients. Although a disciple and initially an admirer of Charcot, Munthe was forced to conclude that almost every theory on the hypnotism preached by Charcot was discarded over time. Munthe wrote:

> To me who for years had been devoting my spare time to study hypnotism, these stage performances of the Salpetriere before the public of tout Paris were nothing but an absurd farce, a hopeless muddle of truth and cheating. Some of these subjects were no doubt real somnambulists faithfully carrying out in a waking state the various suggestions made to them during sleep – post-hypnotic suggestions. Many of them were mere frauds knowing quite well what they were expected to do, delighted to perform their various tricks in public, cheating both doctors and audience with the amazing cunning of the hysteriques.[4]

Munthe believed that the demonstration of hypnotic phenomena should be restricted by law to rare circumstances. When he applied it himself he obtained marvelous results in cases of alcoholism, addiction to morphine and cocaine, and nymphomania, but he admitted that same-sex attachments, which he believed were an acquired deviation from normalcy, were harder to tackle. In addition, he found hypnotic anesthesia to be very effective in alleviating pain after witnessing its effect on dying French soldiers when he spent two days and two nights on the floor of a village church behind the front lines at Verdun during World War I. He acknowledged that a person cannot be hypnotized against his or her will and that all talk about unwilling and unaware individuals being hypnotized at a distance was sheer nonsense, not unlike his view of psychoanalysis.

Dr. Munthe believed that he possessed an exceptional power of which he was aware when he was a boy. He could not only hypnotize successfully nearly all of his patients, but he also could calm and put into lethargy wild animals in a zoo and even charm snakes. Like Dr. Kavorkian, he was never in doubt that the physician must end the misery of animals and humans when the illness was terminal and the suffering unbearable. He describes himself approaching the bedside with his lethal morphine syringe after the old padre had finished the administration of the Last Sacrament. At the same time, he was reluctant to reveal to the dying the gravity of their situation, believing that people do not want to know how ill they are because everyone is afraid of death. He advised physicians to insist on the absolute obedience of the patient, otherwise they must be sent to someone else. He also advised them not to talk too much to patients or they will soon find out how little we know. Doctors, like royalty, must keep aloof as much as possible or their prestige will suffer.

As for women, though they do not seem to know it themselves, he believed that they like to obey far better than to be obeyed. On the whole he thought much better of women than of men but did not admit that to them. Women cannot understand that man is by nature polygamous. They are not less intelligent than men, but their intelligence is of different order. There is no getting beyond the fact that the weight of the man's brain is greater than that of the woman's. He does not believe that women's lesser contributions to art, science and literature result from their lesser exposure, arguing that throughout history women have had the same educational opportunities but have contributed nothing to advance science. All ladies of the Renaissance played some instruments and painted, but there are no great women composers and painters. In today's parlance Axel Munthe is a male chauvinist of the first order who owed a good deal of his reputation as a fashionable doctor to neurotic women treated for imaginary chronic ailments, called sometimes appendicitis and sometimes colitis. The most correct diagnosis ever made by him in those days was overeating, but nobody liked it.

He described himself as a successful doctor whose secret was to inspire confidence, which cannot be acquired by reading or bedside experience. He believed it was a magic gift granted by birthright to one man and denied to another. The doctor who possesses such a gift can almost raise the dead, but one without it will have to call a colleague for consultation in the simplest case of measles. He realized better than anyone that the gifts of his charm and good looks made him a fashionable doctor, but it was important not to become a bad doctor by being too busy to listen to his patients and being indifferent or insensitive to human suffering, an attitude he observed among some pleasure-seeking colleagues. He believed that one cannot be a good doctor without feeling pity, which he possessed in abundance, exhibiting it during epidemics of typhoid fever and diphtheria and, particularly, a cholera epidemic that was killing more than 1000 people a day in Naples in 1910.

Munthe also attended the victims of a catastrophic earthquake in Messina, which killed 60,000 people on December 28, 1908. His idol was Louis Pasteur, who at that time was working on a vaccine for rabies but failed to save six Russian peasants sent to Paris after they had been bitten by a pack of mad wolves.

Many of Munthe's professional colleagues in both capitals were described as greedy and unethical, requesting payment in advance, splitting fees, performing unnecessary surgery and giving useless or dangerous medication. In one case, he prevented the injection of an excessive dose of digitalis that would have killed the patient.

One of the successful physicians used a method of putting healthy neurotics to bed and letting them slowly recover by gradually lifting the imposed restrictions. (Thomas Mann in *The Magic Mountain* had suspected doctors of such practices in the TB sanatorium.) But Munthe admitted that little can be accomplished for hysterical patients outside the hospital.

> You can stun their nerve centers with sedatives but you can not cure them. They remain what they are – a bewildering complex of mental and physical disorders, a plague to themselves and their families and a curse to their doctors.[5]

Among Axel Munthe's reminiscences, the practice of medicine serves as a background for a string of dramatic adventures that are mostly hazardous or improbable, showing him off as a conquering hero. In the preface to the 1936 edition, Munthe himself admitted to having an uncanny feeling that he came out of this book a far better man that he had been in life.

It is hard to remember what attracted the co-author as a medical student to these stories, told by a wild-eyed egomaniac whose escapades are not always credible. It might have been the beautiful prose or a peculiar blend of cynicism and romanticism in a physician whose fees from rich patients allowed him to build the magnificent villa on the most beautiful island in the world and inspired him to tell how he lived there.

## AXEL MUNTHE'S OFFICIAL BIOGRAPHY

Axel Martin Fredrik Munthe was born in 1857 in Oskarshamn, Sweden, and died in 1949 in Stockholm. He was an international figure who spoke several languages: Swedish, English, French, Neapolitan Italian, Capriote Italian and German. He attended medical school in Paris, where he opened his first practice, but later spent most of his adult life in Italy. He was a philanthropist, often treating the poor without charge, and he risked his life on several occasions to help in times of war, disaster or plague, when he could have remained at a safe distance. He was a tireless advocate of animal rights, purchasing land to create a bird sanctuary near his home in Italy and keeping numerous pets as diverse as an owl and a baboon.

In 1887, he moved to Capri, managed to purchase the Villa San Michele and began restoring it, doing much of the work himself. In 1890, running low on money for the renovation, he opened a practice in Rome which catered to foreign dignitaries as well as the local population. From this point on he split his time between Rome and Capri. In 1892 Munthe was appointed physician to the Swedish royal family, and Queen Victoria of Sweden visited him often at the Villa San Michele. In 1907 he married a wealthy English aristocrat, Hilda Pennington-Mellor, and they had two sons. During World War I he served in an ambulance corps and wrote *Red Cross, Iron Cross* about his wartime experiences. In 1929 he published *The Story of San Michele*, which was translated into at least 45 languages and was said to be one of the best-selling books of the 20th century. He spent the final years of his life as an official guest of the King of Sweden.

Munthe willed Villa San Michele to the Swedish nation. It functions as a cultural center maintained by a Swedish foundation, which also supports the Munthe museum and bird sanctuary.[6]

## DOTTORESSA MOOR

The memoirs of the lady doctor Elisabeth Moor cover a long period, spanning her early childhood until her retirement from 40 years of practice in the fishing village of Anacapri on the island of Capri. This locale provides her with an interesting mix of patients: the natives, the tourists during the season and the resident celebrities, among them such writers as Norman Douglas, Compton Mackenzie, Axel Munthe and the editor of the book, the arch-sinner Graham Greene. It is implicit that during this long professional life the Dottoressa set many fractures, sutured many wounds, delivered many babies, dispensed many medicines and comforted many of the dying, but none of this surfaces from the recollected memories of her turbulent life, recorded at the age of 77, when she was half-blind and no longer able to practice. The recording of these memories was urged on her by friends, probably to give her an opportunity to relive some of the episodes in her life and partly to distract her from melancholy. She dictated them in German, with Kenneth MacPherson translating the work into English. When MacPherson died in mid-course, Graham Greene picked up the translation and added some of his own accounts. His editing has preserved the spontaneity without an attempt to erect even a small pedestal for the narrator. With a childlike impishness she recollects various incidents made to appear shocking and outrageous, probably more with the purpose of teasing the reader than of baring her own true soul.

In his preface Graham Greene comments on her forceful vitality, reporting that she was nearly 70 when the last of her uncountable affairs broke up. She bemoaned her inability to live without having someone to love deeply. To grow very old, she says, is to enter the region of death without dying. The recording of memories gives her an opportunity to impart some coherence to the emotional flashbacks lingering within her fading memory. That she makes so little use of it is not because the emotions lacked depth but because, not being an artist, she could not prevent their crumbling into fragments of elementary banality inherent in the prose of daily life.

For a daughter of the Austrian emperor's hairdresser, born in 1885 in Vienna, the prophecy of a career in medicine would have been a most unrealistic scenario, requiring not only a rare talent and a strong determination, but also, most of all, a rebellious spirit. She possessed all of these in abundance, and from early childhood she was bent on defying convention at home and at the convent school, as well as in her early career as a teacher in a language school. After passing the Matura examination at age 20, she declared her wish to study medicine, considered a scandalous profession for a girl from a middle-class family. She was one of only two women admitted to the medical school, the other being her Jewish girlfriend, whose cousin was one of her first lovers. Her desperate parents summoned a well-positioned uncle to persuade her to give up medicine, which he attempted to do by administering a hard beating, without success.

Her memories from medical school recall more lovers than courses. At the age of 24 she was deeply in love with an 18-year-old Swiss painter, Gigi Moor, whom she subsequently married in Geneva shortly before obtaining her medical degree in General Practice. This gave her an opportunity to assist during operations and give anesthesia during World War I. She gave birth to a son, but she and her husband maintained an open-style marriage, with Gigi having an affair with a German cellist and our heroine falling madly in love with a Russian tenor. Elisabeth always boasted that a woman cannot know what real love is if she has not made love with a Russian. The ubiquitous double standard invaded this unconventional household when Gigi, while continuing his affair with the cellist, beat Elisabeth nearly to death when she came home after a night spent with her lover. This was neither the first nor last beating applied to the tough hide of this spirited lady.

After the war she had another child with Gigi in Switzerland, and they subsequently moved to Italy. Her emotional needs seemed satiated by the two children and many lovers, while her marriage dissolved. Italy became her home as she passed an examination for an Italian M.D. degree and received her diploma in 1922 in Pisa. She was pregnant again, unsure who the father was, but certain it was not her husband as they had been separated for some time. After the divorce she left her first-born son with her in-laws in Switzerland and arrived at Capri, her favorite place from previous visits. She was poor as a beggar, with two barefoot children, one dress and nothing else, not even underwear. But the license to practice medicine assured her independence. Most of her patients were poor and she refused to let them pay her, so she worked hard and earned little.

The details of her practice are sketchy, as she preferred to reminisce about her lovers, but it is doubtful whether she could have acquired so much professional recognition and admiration, always difficult to write about in one's own autobiography, without exhibiting medical skill, dogged dedication and empathy. There is no doubt that as a physician she was very much in demand among the locals and foreign expatriates. Her memories impart an image of selflessness, strict adherence to a self-imposed ethical code and fearless courage. Once, attending a child with diphtheria with an Italian doctor who attempted an unsuccessful tracheotomy, during which the child died, she saw the crazed peasant father pulling out a knife and, jumping on her colleague, she grabbed the peasant's wrist near the knife handle and held it until the other doctor ducked out the door. On another occasion she found herself with the stillborn child of an unwed waitress, who begged her to keep the secret of the birth. Elisabeth, after delivering the placenta, hid the child in her big bag and buried the corpse under an orange tree in her garden. She knew that as a doctor she should have reported the birth, but what mattered to her was to be at peace with her God.

During World War II she practiced in Switzerland, but as soon as the war was over, she was on the second train from Switzerland to Italy with her youngest son, a black cocker spaniel and three suitcases. She repossessed her old house and was back in practice in Capri. Her life was nearly shattered by the death of her youngest son and, three years later, by a fatal accident involving her favorite grandson in Switzerland. This was the time when she was urged to write these *Memoirs*, shortly before her departure from Capri, where she could no longer care for herself. She lingered for some time and died at age 90 in 1975, but not before witnessing the publication of her book.

Why should one care about the memories of an egotistic "impossible woman" whose life was so disorderly? Graham Greene offers no particular explanation except his own admiration for this small square creature with blue eyes that would be at home in the windows of the cathedral of Chartres, the big teeth and the wild electric hair as alive as a bundle of fighting snakes. His admiration might have been born at the bedside of many mutual friends dying by their own hand or from disease during his 28-year sojourn on the island of Capri. Or perhaps it was because he saw a woman who was tough and demanding, though frequently self-pitying and bullying her patients. But when she departed, she left a big emptiness among the peasants and the fishermen of the island.

There are not many women physicians in literature. She might not have become a heroic figure if not for the coincidence of living among writers. Her profession of medicine was not a vocation, but rather a rebellion against established customs, a challenge to conformity and, later, a means of making a living and maintaining independence. This is why she is a rare female doctor rivaling in charm and endurance the male characters in the genre of *Zorba the Greek*.

## REFERENCES

1 Munthe A (1929). *The Story of San Michele*. New York: Carroll & Graf; 1991.
2 Moor, E. *An Impossible Woman: The Memoirs of Dottoressa Moor*, edited with an epilogue by Graham Greene. London: Bodley Head; 1975.
3 Wikipedia. *The Story of San Michele*. Available at: http://en.wikipedia.org/wiki/The_Story_of_San_Michele
4 Munthe, op. cit., p. 218.
5 Ibid., p. 237.
6 Wikipedia. *Axel Munthe*. Available at: http://en.wikipedia.org/wiki/Axel_Munthe

# CHAPTER 9

# Dr. Bernard Rieux

## in *The Plague*
### by Albert Camus[1]

---

### Themes

- ■ Existentialism
- ■ Plague as a metaphor for society under attack by an evil force
- ■ Strength and courage of the physicians facing the plague
- ■ When confronted with disaster, there is more to admire in mankind than to despise

---

Albert Camus was a French existentialist novelist and essayist. An acknowledged master of French prose, he embodied the conscience of his times. The essence of existentialism as formulated by J.P. Sartre and Camus is that life has no God-given purpose but is shaped by man's choices and struggles. However, he considered himself more a moralist than a philosopher, an advocate of an atheistic humanism, pointing out the failure of Marxist doctrine and condemning the terror imposed by Communist and Fascist leaders.

He was born in Mondovi, Algeria, to a working-class family. His mother was an illiterate cleaning woman of Spanish extraction; his father, an itinerant agricultural laborer, died in the Battle of the Marne in 1914, when Camus was less than a year old. He grew up poor in the Belcourt section of Algiers but won a scholarship in 1923 to the University of Algiers, where he studied philosophy from 1924 to 1932. Taking time off due to incipient tuberculosis, he held various jobs in Algiers. In 1936 he presented his thesis on Plotinus and received his *diplôme d'études supérieures*, roughly equivalent to an American M.A. After a brief flirtation with the Algerian Communist Party, he became an anarchist and wrote for various anarchist publications, later writing for *Paris-Soir*. He divorced his first wife, Simone Hie, in 1939 and, though he dismissed the institution of marriage as unnatural, a year later married Francine Faure, a pianist and mathematician, with whom he had twins.[2]

The germination of his unique individualism can be seen in the posthumously published notes about his boyhood in a book called *The First Man*. During World War II he moved to Paris, where he participated actively in the anti-German resistance and wrote his first novel, *The Stranger*, and a subsequent essay, *The Myth of Sisyphus*. In these, Camus explored the notion of life's futility, which he dubbed the absurd – the confrontation with ourselves, with our demands for rationality and justice in an indifferent world.

Camus believed that we live in a universe devoid of illusions, where man feels a stranger without hope of a promised land. This divorce between man and his life, like the divorce between the actor and his setting, creates the feeling of absurdity. One can interpret this to mean that, without belief in God or an afterlife, and when suicide is not an option, man develops his own scale of moral values in conformity with the established rules of society. However, the anti-hero in *The Stranger* unconsciously accepts the absurdity of life without any restraints imposed by common sense or intrinsic morality. Absurdity is further explored in *The Plague*, which can be perceived as a metaphor for suffering imposed by forces beyond human control, and this work continues to promote the idea that life is irrational. Furthermore, because it was written in 1947, right after World War II, it is seen by many as representing the evil force of Nazism.

In his last complete novel, *The Fall*,[3] the hero, Jean-Baptiste Clamence, a successful lawyer in Paris, retires to a seedy bar in Amsterdam to peel off the veneer from the surface of his failed life and expose its futility in a confessional monolog. He admits that he was, for more than 30 years, in love exclusively with himself, with women and alcohol providing the only solace. He knew his failings and regretted them but continued to disregard them. On occasion, he pretended to take life seriously, playing at being efficient, indulgent and edifying without ever being sincere and enthusiastic. He had no idea what tasks to accomplish. Clamence extends his experience to all humans – "We are all odd wretched creatures who cannot assert the innocence of anyone whereas we can state with certainty guilt of all."[4]

One wonders where Camus was heading. The only difference between Mersault, the hero of *The Stranger*, and Clamence in *The Fall* is the element of confession, hence insight and remorse, in the latter. In *The Plague*, written before *The Fall*, the narrator of the epidemic, Dr. Rieux, is a strong, courageous man with a clearly defined sense of purpose. Does this mean that the nobility of man can emerge only in the face of adversity?

Camus won the Nobel Prize in Literature in 1957 and died in an automobile accident three years later.

## THE NOVEL

The plague bacillus was first isolated in 1894 by a French bacteriologist, André Yersin, thus the name *Yersinia pestis*. Many outbreaks of plague have caused death and population reduction throughout history. It is believed to have originated in China, but the most famous episode was the notorious Black Death of medieval times, which killed one third of the population of 14th-century Europe. The horrible epidemic caused riots, the displacement of people and, in Germany and Switzerland, persecution of Jews, falsely accused of deliberately poisoning the drinking water. People wandered all over Europe trying to flee the epidemic. Wealth was also displaced as people died and their heirs took over. Newly rich people erected statues and sculptures in cathedrals as signs of gratitude for being spared by the plague. Those who survived believed that there was something special about them, as if God had protected them.

The plague bacillus is transmitted from a carrier, in this case the rat, to a human by a vector, which in the large pandemic of the Middle Ages was the oriental rat flea. The disease appeared in three forms – bubonic, pneumonic and septicemic. The bubonic and septicemic forms were transmitted by direct contact with a flea, while the pneumonic form was transmitted through airborne droplets of saliva coughed up by bubonic or septicemic humans. The incubation time is usually two to six days. In the bubonic type, painfully swelling lymph nodes called buboes appear in the groin and armpits, which ooze pus and blood. The bleeding under the skin causes black blotches. The mortality in untreated cases of bubonic plague is 40% to 60%, but in the other forms it is nearly 100%.

In the novel by Camus the epidemic occurs before effective antibiotics were discovered. It was known, however, that hygienic measures would be adequate to contain an epidemic on the scale pictured in this novel.

Camus was 35 when he wrote *The Plague* in 1947. It was acclaimed as one of the greatest novels of the post-World War II period. It is the story of an outbreak of bubonic plague that takes place in 1940 in the Algerian port of Oran while Algeria was still part of France. Oran, a city of 200,000 people, is immediately isolated from the rest of the world by quarantine and becomes a prison camp or ghetto in which, for almost an entire year, 100 people die each day. The suffering, the despair, the torments of the dying and the survivors, the deprivations, the false hopes, the self-delusions, the lack of restraint and the loss of moral scruples are counterbalanced by greater closeness to loved ones, elimination of social barriers among people facing the same danger and emerging acts of heroism by ordinary men, all recorded by the 35-year-old Dr. Bernard Rieux.

From a medical point of view the story is not very probable. For example, the reason for not allowing any supplies or merchandise into the city is not obvious. But the story works well as an allegory of a society overwhelmed by monstrous calamity and exposed to sociological dissection. Camus describes the paradoxical metamorphoses of active men made indifferent and apathetic and lonesome egoists springing into action with a desire to help.

The most admirable person is Dr. Rieux, the dispassionate recorder of the epidemic's history. The following is his description of himself:

> Looks about thirty-five. Moderate height, broad shoulders, almost rectangular face. Dark steady eyes, but prominent jaws. A biggish, well-modeled nose. Black hair, cropped very close. A curving mouth with thick, usually tight-set lips. He walks quickly. He is absent-minded, when driving his car, often leaves his side-signals on after he has turned a corner. Always bareheaded. Looks knowledgeable.[5]

The epidemic begins with the emergence of thousands of dying rats on the streets of the city and then spreads to the human population. The event does not surprise the narrator, who understands that everyone knows that pestilences have a way of recurring in the world, yet sometimes people find hard to believe the ones that crash down on their heads out of the blue. There have been as many plagues as wars in history, yet always plagues and wars take people equally by surprise.

The plague bacillus is isolated from a swollen lymph node, revealing the nature of the disease. Each day the death toll rises; the quarantine does not check the progress of the epidemic, which leaves the medical profession nearly helpless. For the population, the quarantine has other consequences, such as closing the gates of the city.

> The sudden deprivation befalling people who were completely unprepared for it. Mothers and children, lovers, husbands and wives, who had, a few days previously, taken it for granted that their parting would be a short one, who had kissed one another good-bye on the platform and exchanged a few trivial remarks, sure as they were of seeing one another again after a few days or, at most, a few weeks, duped by our blind human faith in the near future and little if at all diverted from their normal interests by this leave-taking – all these people found themselves, without the least warning, hopelessly cut off,

prevented from seeing one another again, or even communicating with one another.[6]

Dr. Rieux isolated the sick, incised the buboes and waited for the anti-plague serum to arrive, though it turned out not to be very helpful when finally available. Even when one of the other physicians managed to prepare fresh serum against the organism isolated from a patient, it was not clear that this serum worked because, by that time, the plague was close to spending its fury and running its course. By then the hungry monster had satisfied his appetite for killing and was ready to return to his hideout until the next time he struck.

While the epidemic was rampant, however, it was necessary to convert schools and other public buildings to auxiliary hospitals. Camus describes this:

> The floor had been excavated and replaced by a lake of water and cresylic acid, in the center of which was a sort of island made of bricks. The patient was carried to the island, rapidly undressed, and his clothes dropped into the disinfectant water. After being washed, dried and dressed into one of the coarse hospital nightshirts, he was taken to Rieux for examination, then carried to one of the wards. This hospital, a requisitioned schoolhouse, now contained 500 beds, almost all of which were occupied. After the reception of patients, which he personally supervised, Rieux injected serum, lanced buboes, checked the statistics again, and returned for his afternoon consultations. Only when night was setting in did he start on his rounds of visits, and he never got home till a very late hour.[7]

> Rieux had learned that he no longer needed to steel himself against pity. One grows out of pity when it is useless. And in this feeling that his heart had slowly closed in on itself, the doctor found a solace, his only solace for the almost unendurable burden of his days. This he knew would make his task easier, and therefore he was glad of it.[8]

For the entire duration of the epidemic Rieux allowed himself no more than four hours of sleep; he was exhausted to the limit of endurance:

> his sensibility was getting out of hand. Kept under all the time it had grown hard and brittle and seemed to snap completely now and then, leaving him the prey of his emotions . . . he had few illusions left, and fatigue was robbing him of even those remaining few. He knew that over a period whose end he

could not glimpse, his task was no longer to cure but diagnose. He felt that he was not dispensing medical help but only information. In this he felt that his exhaustion was a blessing. Had he been less tired, his senses more alert, that all-pervading odor of death might have made him sentimental. But when a man has only four hours of sleep he is not sentimental. He sees things as they are; that is to say, he sees them in the garish light of justice – hideous witless justice. He regrets that the epidemic transforms him from a man welcomed by his patients as a healer and savior into a feared executor of separation, breaking into apartments with soldiers to drag away the sick person to the hospital and quarantine the rest of the family.[9]

Dr. Rieux is not a believer but, when invited by his friend, the scholarly Jesuit priest Father Paneloux, he comes to church to listen to Paneloux's sermons. Early in the epidemic Father Paneloux preaches to his parishioners that God sent the plague to punish the sinners and unbelievers, likening it to the punishment of Sodom and Gomorrah in the Bible. Later, however, when Father Paneloux joins Rieux's band of workers in the hospital and witnesses the suffering of patients, he acknowledges that his earlier words and thoughts lacked charity, and even though we do not understand God's will, we have only the love of Him to reconcile us with suffering and the death of children. Dr. Rieux thinks that the later sermon displays more uneasiness than real power.

Another friend who has much in common with Dr. Rieux is Jean Tarrou, a visitor trapped in the city by the quarantine. Observing that the sanitary department is understaffed and inefficient, he draws up a plan to organize groups of voluntary helpers, which the doctor gratefully accepts.

Tarrou asks Dr. Rieux, "Why do you yourself show such devotion, considering you don't believe in God?"

Dr. Rieux answers that his profession is to cure sick people. Moreover, he never managed to get used seeing people die, but

> "since the order of the world is shaped by death, mightn't it be better for God if we refuse to believe in Him and struggle with all our might against death, without raising our eyes toward the heavens where He sits in silence?"
>
> "Who taught you all this, Doctor?" asks Tarrou.
>
> The reply comes promptly. "Suffering."

When, in turn, Tarrou is asked the same question, he answers

> "I do not know. My code of morals, perhaps."
>
> "What code is that?"

The answer is "Comprehension," and later, "All I maintain is that on this earth there are pestilences and there are victims, and it is up to us as far as possible not to join forces with the pestilences."[10]

Unlike many of his friends and assistants, including Tarrou and Father Paneloux, Dr. Rieux survives the epidemic of plague. His wife, who had been sent to a tuberculosis sanatorium before the outbreak, dies there, but he's comforted by his loving mother. Rieux is a lone human being who emerges from a nightmarish experience with a clearer vision of humanity. He learns from the time of the pestilence that there are more things to admire in men than to despise.

## REFERENCES

1  Camus A (1947). *The Plague*. Translated from the French by S Gilbert. New York: Alfred A Knopf; 1948.
2  Wikipedia. *Albert Camus*. Available at: http://en.wikipedia.org/wiki/Albert_Camus; Liukkonen P. *Albert Camus (1913–1960)*. Available at: www.kirjasto.sci.fi/acamus.htm
3  Camus A (1956). *The Fall*. Translated from the French by J O'Brien. New York: Vintage International; 1991.
4  Ibid., p. 110.
5  Camus, op. cit., *The Plague*. p. 27.
6  Ibid., p. 61.
7  Ibid., p. 81.
8  Ibid., p. 83.
9  Ibid., p. 172.
10  Ibid., from dialogue on pp. 116–20.

## PART THREE

# Destroyed careers

# CHAPTER 10

# Dr. Antoine Thibault

## in *Les Thibault*

### by Roger Martin du Gard[1]

---

### Themes

- Catholic-Protestant split and atheism in early 20th-century France
- Intense but doomed love affair transforms the doctor's personality
- Medical practice and the morality of euthanasia
- A generation of young men killed and maimed in the trenches of World War I
- Prophecy of World War II

---

Roger Martin du Gard came from a prosperous and intellectual background. His father was a lawyer and his mother's family were stockbrokers. When he was 17 years old he read Tolstoy's *War and Peace*, which was an inspiration for the Thibault saga. Another influential book might have been *The Brothers Karamazov* by Dostoyevsky. Educated at the École des Chartres in Paris, he graduated as a paleographer (who studies and interprets ancient documents) and archivist in 1905. He self-published his first novel, *Devenir*, in 1907, but it was not until 1913 that his major breakthrough came with *Jean Barois*, a fictional account of the Dreyfuss affair, which André Gide recommended to his publisher. Martin Du Gard served in the French army in a motor transport division during World War I; afterwards he retired to Le Tertre, a country estate in Normandy, where he wrote *Les Thibault*, a family saga released in eight installments of varying length between 1922 and 1940. His final work, *Le Lieutenant-Colonel Maumort*, remained unfinished at his death in 1958.

## THE NOVEL

*Les Thibault*, for which Roger Martin du Gard was awarded the Nobel Prize in Literature in 1937, covers the history of two upper-middle-class families in Paris in the years between 1905 and 1918, the Thibaults of the title, prosperous, conservative and Catholic, and the de Fontanins, cash poor, liberal and Protestant. The vast chronicle explores the social and moral issues confronting the French bourgeoisie during the early 20th century. The Thibault family is represented by the father, Oscar, and two sons, a 25-year-old physician, Antoine, and his 15-year-old brother, Jacques. Oscar Thibault is a retired lawyer – a pious Catholic intolerant of Protestants and a strict disciplinarian who, at the onset of the novel, is set to punish the rebellious Jacques for rejecting the established order and later turning to revolutionary socialism.

Antoine, the most sympathetic of the Thibaults, remains determined to protect his brother from their father's ire. He does not reject his bourgeois heritage but abandons the Catholic faith instilled in him during childhood. Of the de Fontanin family, the lives of two children, Daniel and Jenny, intersect with those of the Thibault brothers. The novel was uniformly praised for its objectivity and scrupulous regard for detail, which apply to the images of medical practice, the main theme of the following discussion.

The first medical episode in the book deals with the illness of the sensitive 12-year-old Jenny de Fontanin, who contracts meningitis and, according to all her doctors – including Antoine Thibault – is dying. Mme. de Fontanin is alone to deal with this crisis, as her philandering husband has disappeared and her son Daniel has run away from home with Jacques Thibault, which is why Antoine appears on the scene. She summons her old friend, Pastor James Gregory, a tall, ungainly, grotesquely thin man, who orders her to send the doctors away and prays over the prostrate child. A believer in healing prayer, which chases out evil, the source of all illness, Pastor Gregory is thus an early 20th-century alternative healer and a successful one, since Jenny survives.

Dr. Antoine Thibault, house physician at the Children's Hospital, is a rationalist with a quick, retentive mind. He is industrious, ambitious, self-reliant and fond of challenges, and he has chosen to specialize in children's diseases because with children one can count only on oneself. He is assistant to the noted Dr. Philip and is in love with medicine, calling it a

> "career worthy of a Thibault. Hard, I grant you, but how rewarding, when one has a taste for fighting against odds, and a bit of personal pride. Think of all the attention, memory, willpower it demands! . . . And consider what it means when one's made good! A great doctor, that's somebody! A Philip, for instance.

One has to learn, of course, how to adopt that gentle, assured manner. Very courteous, but distant."[2]

But Antoine can be rancorous. He is defiant when Dr. Philip corrects him in front of colleagues for misdiagnosing a case of infantile diabetes and longs to point out that, if the chief came in early and didn't run off to see his paying patients, Antoine would not have to attend to Philip's hospital cases and would have had more time to examine his own patients without missing important clues. At the same time Antoine admires and envies Philip, who has amazing intuition. He questions his own future. "Shall I ever get to understand things in a flash, as he does? Shall I ever have that almost infallible perspicacity which is what really makes the great physician?"[3]

Much later, in his diary written during his terminal illness, Antoine confesses to his vanity and his desire for approval and admiration from the younger doctors. He believes that his diagnostic performance was better in the hospital in the presence of colleagues than when alone in the office.

Physically, Antoine has a large head, a thick beard and a bulging forehead and he cultivates a look of grim determination, but Mme. de Fontanin admires him immensely:

> Antoine came in with a firm, decided step, now that he had accepted all the consequences this visit might entail. The light from the open windows fell full on his face; his hair and beard formed zones of shadow and all the sunlight seemed concentrated on the pale rectangle of his forehead, lending him an air of high intellectuality. And, though he was of medium height, at that moment he seemed tall.[4]

Dr. Thibault's working days are so long that he hardly goes out at night. Women don't matter much, except for occasional visits to cafés and casual adventures with prostitutes. But things change when he falls in love. This happens when his assistant's child, Dédette, is run over by a car. Antoine rushes to their house and finds a critically injured young girl in shock, with a fractured femur and profuse bleeding from the femoral artery. Using his suspenders as a tourniquet to stop the bleeding, he operates at once. A local doctor helps him and he presses into service a beautiful young woman in a pink dressing gown who happens to be there. The proverbial kitchen table serves to hold the dying child; an ordinary lamp with its shade removed lights the operating field; a side table holds his instruments – scalpel, forceps, gauze, cotton-wool, alcohol, caffeine, tincture of iodine. Antoine lays a series of compresses around the wound and proceeds with the incision. He repairs the artery using plaited silk, closes, bandages, removes the tourniquet. Dédette's pulse is so rapid it is beyond counting. Antoine sends the mysterious young woman in pink to the pharmacy for saline and orders his assistant to inject camphor first, then caffeine. When the woman returns he rigs up an IV, using a Swiss wall barometer and looping the rubber tubing around a saucepan filled with hot water to warm the saline solution as it flows through, then lays bare a vein in the child's arm with his scalpel and inserts the needle. Ten tense minutes pass: the pulse becomes palpable at 140 beats and her breathing is easier. Antoine experiences huge relief. "It was all he could do to stay where he was; he had a childish longing to sing or whistle."[5] After he sets the leg, he rigs up a pulley with string, using a flatiron as a counterweight to stretch it.

The encounter with the woman in the pink dressing gown, who attracted his interest in the midst of the surgical turmoil, marks the beginning of the great love of his life. Soon his doctoring recedes to the background as he becomes more and more obsessed with Rachel Goepert, a woman with a history (in French avanturière) – many affairs, a child who died, and her lover, Hirsch, a major influence in her life, who, though cruel, and described in French as a mysterious bandit, fascinates her, keeps her in a sort of unwilling but unbreakable bondage and takes her to Africa, where she falls under the spell of the "dark continent."

Antoine recognizes their profound differences, but by inflaming his passion, she transforms him deeply, both externally and internally. He shaves off his beard, which "exposed a light hollow in the cheeks – a certain slackness of the tissues – giving them a milder air that somewhat redeemed the sternness of the jaw. But it also exposed the long, sinuous line of his mouth,"[6] which connotes to her more than human willpower. Antoine acknowledges deeper changes: his temperament has softened and he has become more mature yet somehow younger. He thinks he has gained strength of mind; that he is both more forceful and more spontaneous.

The affair is doomed; despite her deep love for Antoine, Rachel leaves him to marry Hirsch and join him in Africa. There is a poignant farewell, one of the great goodbyes in literature, with Antoine standing alone in the rain on the far end of the northern jetty at Le Havre, near the foot of the lighthouse, surrounded by a wild turmoil of wind and waves, with streaks of livid light accompanying the dawn, watching the ship that is taking away his love. In the empty station waiting room, early for the train that will take him back to Paris, he falls into a trance, imagining Rachel in his arms once more, and thinks of suicide. But in his regained solitude, Antoine chooses a different path. He dedicates himself with passion to being of service to humanity, represented by his office patients, varying in class, education and ability to pay. The practice grows and the work distracts him from his grief.

There are instances of serious ethical dilemmas. The intractable pain of a child with an incurable disease calls for morphine, but he refuses to give a larger dose that would result in euthanasia. He claims the sanctity of human life even as he admits to himself that there is no sense in all this pain. After refusing to double the dose, he leaves but worries that his assistant will do it and he'll be blamed. Worse, he realizes he acted against his own beliefs. He remembers that when he was 16 and the family was vacationing in Brittany, there was a case of a child with two heads whose father tried to kill it when the doctor refused, and that he had a violent argument with his own father over his certainty that a doctor should be allowed to cut short a doomed life. This musing over morality goes on for several pages until Antoine finally admits that he's still a mystery to himself and wonders if he will ever know what his guiding principle is. Later, in his terminal diary, he compares his actions driven by an impulse with the decisions dictated by reason and concludes that the most important judgments in his life were made spontaneously.

Finally, we arrive at the great medical spectacle of the novel – the long, drawn-out, horrible death from uremia suffered by Oscar Thibault. We start with the business of lying to the patient. After the old man cries that he's going to die, Antoine believes that it is imperative to root out immediately the least trace of suspicion from the patient's mind. He makes a big fuss about changing the serum he's injecting, trying to use the power of suggestion to make his father feel better, even as he knows that the illness is incurable. He succeeds in fooling his father that the new medication is better, though it is the same. Then he smugly says to himself, "I'm getting smarter at this sort of thing every day."[7] It seems doctors have long been aware of the placebo effect. Meanwhile, the condition of the patient worsens.

Antoine learns that his brother Jacques has become a journalist, writer and political activist involved with the international socialist movement in Switzerland. He travels there to bring him home before their father dies. They arrive to find that the old man's kidneys have failed completely and think the end is near. But one kidney resumes function spontaneously, which does not stop the pain. The morphine injections have been discontinued because they could kill the patient. The question of euthanasia reappears; Antoine's colleague, Therivier, reads this question in Antoine's eyes and understands what he wants but admonishes him that we aren't murderers. This misery goes on for several days and through 34 pages. Jacques appeals to his doctor brother to do something, as the father's agonizing screams keep rising. Critics have repeatedly called this portion of the novel the most effective (and accurate) death scene ever written.

Still alive at midnight, the father suffers attacks of pain that come in quick succession. Antoine waits for the next one as he watches his father's suffering.

> It promised to be catastrophic; all the usual symptoms were present, but in a hideously intensified form. The breathing had nearly stopped, the face was congested, the eyes were starting from their sockets, the forearms tensely contracted and flexed so sharply that the hands were hidden and the wrists, folded beneath the beard, had the look of amputated stumps. All the limbs were quivering with the formidable tension, and the sinews seemed on the point of snapping under the strain. Never before had the phase of rigidity lasted so long; the seconds went by and it showed no sign of easing. Antoine fully believed the end had come.[8]

At one point they send out for oxygen when they see he is suffocating. The ambivalence – praying for death but doing nothing to help it along – is extreme. At last, Antoine, exhausted physically and emotionally, gives his father a shot of morphine. The brothers watch as the drug takes effect: ". . . the features were relaxing, the marks of many days of agony being smoothed away, and the mortal lethargy now settling on the tranquil face might have been the calm of a refreshing sleep."[9]

Still the old man hangs on, through the arrival of the servants and retainers, who kneel around the bed, praying. Finally, the heart stops and Antoine can close his father's eyes. At first he feels no guilt, does not even think much about what he has done. His moral struggles are turned more toward his absence of belief and the question of whether death is really the end. But when Dr. Hequet pays a condolence call, he can no longer avoid the issue of guilt, of right and wrong.

> He understood that the decisive act he had carried out on the previous day in cold blood – an act which he still whole-heartedly commended – was something which he must now assimilate, as it were, with his personality, fit into his scheme of things. It was one of those crucial experiences which have far-reaching influence on the shaping of a man's character; and he felt that his mental centre of gravity would have to be readjusted to meet the stress of this new increment.[10]

It's not entirely clear if this integration takes place. A long conversation between Antoine and the Abbé Vecard, his father's spiritual advisor, as they return from M. Thibault's funeral is a classic wrangle between believer and atheist. As the

Abbé extols the virtues of the Catholic faith, Antoine, calling himself a natural, congenital skeptic, is provoked to reveal his own true belief.

> "My atheism and my mind developed side by side, so I've never had any allegiance to renounce. No, don't imagine for a moment that I'm one of those believers who have lost their faith, and in their hearts are always craving after God; one of those uneasy souls who make desperate gestures toward the heavens they have found empty. No, desperate gestures aren't in my line at all. There's nothing about a godless world that disturbs me; indeed, as you see, I'm perfectly at home in it."[11]

To underline his ideas he tells the Abbé that he feels as far from Catholic mythology as from pagan mythology and claims to make no distinction between religion and superstition. Later in his diary he expands on this subject, claiming that God is a human invention for shifting the burden of good and evil. He rejects the notion that morality is God-given and attributes it to the experiences of humans organizing and regulating the collective life as social animals, to be transmitted from generation to generation by tradition and heredity. No God ever responded to the appeals for intervention of man, he notes. At the end of his life he dismisses the priest coming to perform the last rites. He asks him: What did the church do to prevent the war? You and your German priests blessed the flags and sang "Te Deum" to praise God for the massacres. At the end of the book the author expresses the belief that death is simpler for a non-believer.

Originally, *Les Thibault* ended at this point, but the next installment, Part 5, *L'Été 1914*,[12] was published in 1936; it is this work that the Nobel Committee cited when awarding the Prize.

In this subsequent version, Jacques returns to Switzerland after his father's death and becomes ever more radical and involved with the international socialist movement attempting to prevent the war. Antoine remodels his father's house, sets up a laboratory, employs three researchers and is so engrossed with his ambitious projects and his practice that he is amazed when Jacques appears during the summer to warn him of the approaching war. Jenny arrives to tell the brothers her father is dying after shooting himself in the head while trying to commit suicide; this brings Jacques and Jenny together. When mobilization is announced on August 1, Jacques, who refuses to be called up, leaves for Switzerland, taking Jenny with him. Antoine stoically accepts the disruption of his projects and is mobilized. Jacques conceives a mad idea: to get his colleague Meynestrel, a pilot, to fly him over the front lines, where they will drop pacifist leaflets rallying the soldiers on both sides to resist the propaganda of the ruling class and refuse to fight. He understands it will be a suicide flight but has no wish to live in a world at war.

*L'Été* ends here but Martin du Gard was not yet finished. In his 320-page *Epilogue*, published in 1940,[13] he leaps ahead to May 1918 and deals with Antoine's fate. Antoine was gassed with yperite (mustard gas) in 1917 and suffered from severe damage to his larynx and the rest of his respiratory system. He is at a clinic for gas victims in the south of France, where he follows the treatment of the other patients and keeps careful clinical records of his own symptoms, which he believes to be of possible value to science. He leaves the clinic to attend the funeral of their old housekeeper in Paris and, going through piles of mail, finds the amber necklace he had once given Rachel. Later he learns she died in 1916. He confesses in his diary that this was the best encounter in his poor life. If only he could have died in her arms, he writes.

Antoine visits Dr. Philip and sees in his eyes pity for a doomed man; it is then that he realizes that he will not survive. Dr. Philip (le patron) is bitter. Of his six favorite assistants, who were like his children, three were killed, two disabled, and Antoine is the last. Philip recalls wistfully the peaceful society guided by reason at the end of the 19th century. But, he thinks, we should not have forgotten the dormant human instincts always ready to destroy the constructive forces in nature and to debase the edifying ideas of tolerance – the forces that were unleashed during the past four years in Europe.

Antoine's diary also alludes frequently to the absurdity of the war, which aborted his career and then killed him. He witnessed how war unleashes the brute destructive force, killing, maiming, impoverishing the displaced population and disrupting the social structure. In a moment of introspection he acknowledges that the war did release in him the deeply submerged feelings of hate, violence, fear, cruelty and contempt for the weak. This insight gives him greater understanding of the roots of human vicissitudes and criminality.

At first the unspoken verdict of Patron Philip numbs him; later he tries to reconnect with his world. He offers to marry Jenny and make legitimate the three-year old son of Jacques, Jean-Paul, but she refuses. However, one of his two diaries is written for Jean-Paul, for the time when he grows up. He reminds him to be aware that the man's life is incredibly short and that there will be little time to realize this, but says he believes that at the age of 25 in 1940 he will live in a peaceful reconstructed Europe, no longer plagued by nationalism because the experiences of this war will lead, if not to fraternity, at least to a better understanding among nations. This is probably written with tongue in cheek, because at the time Martin du Guard knew where Europe was heading. Therefore, there is not much prophecy in Antoine's warnings that the success of the peace treaty will depend on our attitude toward the defeated nations and that arms limitation should be equally imposed on the winners and losers. But, unfortunately, the more victorious we feel, the less conciliatory we are and we treat the defeated with greater harshness, thus denying the possibility of a durable reconciliation.

Antoine secures for himself the morphine that will prevent the suffering his father experienced, and then deals with the questions he left unanswered in his debate with the good Abbé. Returning to those questions, he can admit only that all one's actions are in the name of nothing. But he leaves one question open and it is – what is the significance of life, what is it all for? This Antoine fails to answer. He predicts, however, that nothing of him will survive after his death.

This apparently was Roger Martin du Gard's belief. In a letter cited in a book by David L. Schalk,[14] he wrote that man has no preordained or meaningful destiny in this world or any other. Schalk then quotes a passage from the *Epilogue* when Antoine remembers passing the hospital nursery and watching the small patients play with blocks. Some moved them around haphazardly; others sorted them out by color or made geometrical designs; still others tried to build little shaky edifices. Some of the more tenacious would even construct a bridge, an obelisk, even a high pyramid. But when the play period ended, all the blocks were scattered about the floor. This is what life is like; we assemble what we can out of the elements at hand. "The most gifted attempt to make of their lives a complicated construction, a veritable work of art. One must try to be among this group, so that the recreation can be as amusing as possible."[15] Antoine commits suicide on November 18, 1918 at the age of 37 years, four months and nine days. The final notation in his journal is "Jean-Paul."

Thinking of Antoine, the first thing we see is that his love affair with Rachel changes him and allows him to grow. He is a wonderfully tender lover, an exemplary physician, a man of principle and a moralist who does not waiver in his deepest belief even when facing death. He is the most introspective physician immortalized in literature by a non-physician. All the other doctors in this novel – Hequet, Therivier, the awe-struck young neighborhood doctor who helps Antoine save Dédette's life, even the great and impatient Dr. Philip – are also presented in a sympathetic light. If literature tells us anything about an age, it is that, in this period at least, doctors were men of stature commanding respect. But in such a massive work, whose theme is the inadequacy and hopelessness of man, one wonders if Roger Martin du Gard chose medicine as the profession of his main hero to underline his belief that, for the first half of the 20th century, even a healer cannot avoid irrational and self-destructive human behavior. Everyone in this story is doomed: Jenny in permanent mourning for Jacques; Antoine and Jacques dead and the Thibault name obliterated; Daniel only waiting for his mother to die so that he can commit suicide. The most optimistic thing one can derive from this novel is that Roger Martin du Gard has created a remarkable work of fiction in which the tenderness of love, the practice of medicine with all its moral dilemmas, the struggle with the image of God, the inevitability of death and the horrors of war are revealed realistically by a sensitive and sympathetic physician. This is one of the books that without question deserved the Nobel Prize. It is regrettable that the last volume is not available in English translation.

## REFERENCES

1 Martin du Guard R. *Les Thibault.* Paris: Gallimard; 1953.
2 Ibid., p. 190.
3 Ibid., p. 193.
4 Ibid., p. 229.
5 Ibid., p. 326.
6 Ibid., p. 457.
7 Ibid., p. 613.
8 Ibid., p. 615.
9 Ibid., p. 745.
10 Ibid., pp. 769–70.
11 Ibid. pp. 774–5.
12 Martin du Gard R. *Les Thibault V: L'Été 1914 (fin).* Paris: Gallimard; 1967.
13 Martin du Gard R. *Les Thibault V: Epilogue.* Paris: Gallimard; 1967.
14 Schalk DL. *Roger Martin du Gard: the novelist and history.* New York: Cornell University Press; 1967.
15 Ibid., pp. 172–3.

# CHAPTER 11

# Dr. Ravic

## in *Arch of Triumph*
### by Erich Maria Remarque[1]

---

### Themes

- Political refugee from Nazi Germany practices as a ghost surgeon in Paris
- A revenge killing that may be justified homicide
- Victims of illegal abortion

---

Eric Maria Remarque was born in the town of Osnabruck in northwestern Germany, to a family of modest means and French ancestry. His father was a bookbinder. He excelled in school but his studies at the University of Muenster were interrupted when he turned 18 and was conscripted into the army. On June 12, 1917 he was transferred to the Western Front, and at the end of July he was wounded by shrapnel in the left leg, right arm and neck and was repatriated to an army hospital in Germany, where he spent the rest of the war. After the war he changed his last name from Remark to Remarque, which previously had been the family name. He taught school and was a stone cutter and a test car driver. Finally, he became an assistant editor at a sports magazine. In 1929 he published his most famous work, *All Quiet on the Western Front*. The novel, which pictured in understated language the horror of trench warfare from the perspective of a 20-year-old soldier, sold 1.2 million copies in its first year, sparked waves of political controversy and is considered the best novel about World War I by many readers and critics. The sequel, *The Way Back*, appeared in 1931. It dealt with the collapse of the German Army after the war. In 1933 the Nazis banned and burned Remarque's books and issued propaganda that he was a Jew, which is not true, and that he had never seen active service. In 1943 the Nazis arrested his sister, Elfriede, who had stayed in Germany with her husband and two children, and, after a short trial, found her guilty of undermining morality. As her brother was beyond reach, the Nazis sentenced her to death. On a specific order of Adolph Hitler she was decapitated with an axe.[2]

Remarque moved to Switzerland in 1932, and in 1939 he emigrated to the United States, where he became a citizen in 1947. He was a celebrity, hanging out at the Stork Club in New York and, in Hollywood, making friends with Paulette Goddard, whom he married in 1958. He had been married twice before, to the same woman, Jutta Zambona, first in 1925 and again in 1938. He later settled in Switzerland, where he died from an aortic aneurysm in 1970.

Remarque's later works dealt with the European political upheavals from the 1920s to the Cold War. While they did not achieve the fame of his earlier novels, his ability to create interesting plots and memorable characters made them highly popular with readers. His play *Die Letzte Station* (*The Last Station*) was about the fall of the Third Reich; *Spark of Life* was a fictional documentary about Nazi concentration camps; and *The Black Obelisk* dealt with life in the chaotic Germany of the 1920s.

**THE NOVEL**

This potboiler centers on a stateless political refugee, an accomplished surgeon from Germany, Ludwig Fresenburg, who has no legal documents and lives under the assumed name of Ravic in a refugee hideout called the International. The action takes place in Paris in 1939. He has no permission to perform surgery and can only work anonymously as "a ghost surgeon," operating on patients for two less skillful French physicians. He arrives in the operating room masked and gowned after the patient has been anesthetized and leaves before the anesthesia wears off. In Germany he was a hospital department head but, after the Nazi takeover, he was arrested and sent to a concentration camp because he participated in the Spanish Civil War on the side of legitimate government, which was defending the country against an invasion by General Francisco Franco, who was aided by Nazi Germany and Fascist Italy.

Ravic must accept whatever his patron doctors pay him for his skill – apparently enough from good-guy Dr. Veber to buy an endless supply of vodka and calvados (apple brandy) but a mere pittance from the miserly society physician Dr. Durant. Ravic operates with a detached acceptance of his professional demotion, bearing scars from torture inflicted by a Gestapo agent named Haake, commandant of the German concentration camp from which he escaped, leaving behind his lover Sybil, whom Haake tortured and killed because she refused to betray Ravic's hideout.

The war in Spain had taught him a survival philosophy: Help when you can – do everything good then – but when you can no longer do anything, forget it! Leave it and pull yourself together. Compassion, he believed, is meant for quiet times, not when life is at stake. As he, a stateless refugee banished from the orderly society of his former peers and brutalized by imprisonment, undergoes further emotional hardening, he becomes a lonely outcast convinced that nothing any longer can surprise him, living day by day while consoling himself with alcohol and casual liaisons with easily available women. For the people surrounding him, living their orderly undisturbed life, he feels contempt rather than envy.

Ravic has been deported from France a few times and knows it will happen again. In the meantime he loves to operate. He thinks it would be impossible to explain to Dr. Veber – the quintessential bourgeois Frenchman with his perfect doll's house in the suburbs, with a neat woman and two neat children in it – the excitement of "that breathless tension when the knife first cut and the narrow red trace followed the light pressure, when the body, under clips and forceps, opened up like a multiple curtain."[3]

At the root of such sarcasm and veiled contempt is probably the envy of the normal social and professional life granted to a less talented and less competent colleague, who may be unable to understand how frustrated Ravic is by being deprived of direct contact with patients, the acceptance of their gratitude he once was used to and, of course, proper remuneration.

The turgid writing continues but Ravic's surgical successes do not. He fails to save a 21-year-old woman from a botched abortion, because she arrives at Veber's hospital too late. Subsequently he does save her friend, Lucienne, who is in a similar predicament. He dares to confront the female abortionist, Madame Boucher, from whom he tries to obtain a refund for the impoverished girl by threatening to expose her, a silly move since she's a tough old lady who knows at once that he's a vulnerable refugee. Afterwards, Ravic reflects on the consequences of illegal abortion and the misery it causes. Decent Ravic then gives Lucienne 100 francs from his own pocket, lying that Madame Boucher returned it.

One of Ravic's professional sources of income is from examining weekly the girls at the Osiris, a large middle-class brothel, where Rolande is the golden-hearted manager who is engaged in her profession to save enough money to open a restaurant. Another case involves an injured boy who hopes Ravic will not restore the function of his crushed leg because he and his poor old mother will collect more from the insurance and be able to start a business if he's completely disabled. Ravic obliges, but only because the leg is not salvageable.

The first part of the book is taken up with Ravic's affair with Joan Madou, a woman he finds walking dazedly around the deserted streets in the middle of the night. Joan has a good reason to be confused and sad. Her lover has died in their hotel room; she doesn't know a soul in Paris, and being a dependent sort, has no idea what to do. Ravic takes care of everything – gets a French doctor to write the death certificate, calls the police, has the body removed, quiets the hotel keeper, obtains for Joan, who claims to be a mediocre singer and actress, a job at a nightclub and becomes her lover after the few weeks it takes for her to cease mourning. In this affair there are no love declarations; there is only the image of a bed in a dark hotel room with two glowing cigarettes and a flask of apple brandy on the night table. One episode of brief happiness is a trip to the Riviera funded by Ravic, who makes Durant pay him 2000 francs for an operation on a wealthy socialite instead of the usual 200 francs. Joan longs for a stable relationship in their own apartment, failing to understand Ravic's tenuous situation. But fate intervenes when Ravic stops to examine a woman who is lying on the pavement, having been injured by a falling girder at a construction site. Immersed in his examination, he doesn't leave the site fast enough when the gendarmes arrive and discover he has no legal permit to stay in France. By the time he returns from three months' exile in Switzerland, Joan has taken another lover, but shortly afterwards he finds a more important mission and Joan fades from view.

His tormentor, Haake, the Gestapo agent, turns up in Paris on the staff of the German embassy, presumably to spy on the political refugees. Ravic thinks he had seen him a few times earlier in Paris only to have him disappear. In fact, at first, he's sure that he is hallucinating. But finally Ravic finds him eating in a café and engages him in conversation, during which he invites him to a place that sells pornographic pictures. Haake falls for this lure and accompanies Ravic to an uninhabited site, where Ravic kills him with a revolver, buries the body in the woods of St. Germain and burns all the evidence, without a drop of blood spilling on the rental car that he drives without a license. He is never stopped, in spite of speeding, and is released from his years of pain because he has finally avenged Sybil and himself. This is a perfect crime.

Joan's actor lover shoots her accidentally and she dies in Ravic's arms. As the novel ends, war breaks out in Poland; all refugees are rounded up by the French police and Ravic goes off to the French detention camp with his medical kit, knowing that doctors are always useful.

This story was adapted in a film in 1947 staring Charles Boyer and Ingrid Bergman and was also adapted for TV, with Anthony Hopkins as Ravic.

*Arch of Triumph* is not a novel about the practice of medicine, of which

Remarque probably had limited knowledge, but he did know well the plight of refugees from Nazi Germany, and he probably knew Paris, with its Arc de Triomphe, a city that in the years before World War II was the Mecca for writers and artists and a haven for political refugees, beginning with Russian émigrés after the 1918 revolution. Paris was a temporary and in some cases a permanent home for a large number of American writers, among them Gertrude Stein, Ernest Hemingway, James Baldwin, Scott Fitzgerald, Sinclair Lewis and the Russian writers Vladimir Nabokov and Irene Nemirovsky. The life and works of these celebrities were vastly publicized. At the same time, the large cohort of legal and illegal immigrants, particularly those from Hitler's Germany, struggled to survive in obscurity.

Dr. Ravic's story sheds some light on the plight of the stateless immigrant without proper documents who happens to be a highly qualified surgeon. This profession provides him with the means to live modestly and inconspicuously, albeit in fear of being arrested by a suspicious gendarme or of being denounced by an extortionist. It is not surprising that his best friend is a Russian count employed as a doorman in a nightclub, a comrade in the fall from grace. Dr. Ravic has erased all connections to the past and assumed a new identity but has preserved his professional integrity. His heavy drinking and frequent affairs bear a macho stamp, but he is not immune to falling in love or suffering when betrayed by a lover. At the end, we do not know whether he will still be in France after the German invasion, to fall once again into the clutches of the Gestapo, or whether he will have managed to escape to England or a neutral country in Europe.

## REFUGEE PHYSICIANS IN THE UNITED STATES

How would Dr. Ravic have fared if he succeeded in immigrating to the United States? This question can be answered by reading from E.D. Kohler's *Relicensing Central European Refugee Physicians in the United States (1933–1945)*.[4] Between 1933 and 1941, 3097 physicians found sanctuary in the United States from Nazi persecution. The refugee physicians encountered a system of states' rights requirements for a license to practice medicine that was different in each of the 48 states. In 1940 only 15 states accepted foreigners and Americans with foreign medical credentials, but five of those deliberately discouraged such persons from applying. The professional fate of most refugee physicians were determined by bureaucrats who headed the various states' medical licensing boards. During the worst depression in American history, the boards had a vested interest in keeping out potential competitors. Hence they began adopting measures to deny licenses to all foreign medical graduates. Many boards began to demand American citizenship for a medical license, some five years away for most immigrants.

The majority of medical refugees settled in four states – California, Illinois, Ohio and New York. In 1933, the California Board of Medical Examiners began to demand, as prerequisites for granting licenses, that foreign medical graduates obtain licenses from the countries in which they had received their diplomas and also serve a one-year rotating internship in an American Medical Association-approved hospital. For Jewish physicians, obtaining certificates from Germany, Austria and occupied Czechoslovakia was not possible, since the Nazis had revoked their licenses.

In California these ploys had other effects on the physician refugees. The rotating internship requirement, which involved a year of uncompensated work, made qualification for a license a luxury few could afford. Accordingly, a count of identifiable refugee physicians in the California section of the 1950 *American Medical Directory* shows only 175 German and Austrian degree holders, about 1% of physicians in the state.

In Ohio, the State Medical Society sought to discourage refugee physicians by demanding additional course work in American history, civics and college English, subjects obviously not included in European premedical studies. Another Ohio ploy was to refuse licenses to foreign-trained physicians on the ground that the countries where their degrees had been earned would not license Ohio-trained physicians.

New York was the state that never closed its doors, and more than two-thirds of the medical refugees settled there. The expatriate physicians had to face written and oral examination testing their competency in English, as well as the nation's toughest four-day written medical examination. It was thus not surprising that the initial failure rate was 70% and higher. Inability to pass the examination frequently forced a significant number of refugee physicians to work at menial jobs – dishwashing and waiting tables – before taking the examination again. As in California, the physicians' wives often kept food on the family table by working at unskilled or semi-skilled jobs, while the doctors studied for the difficult re-examination in one of the few states left in the country in which they could be re-licensed to practice. On balance, however, the states that accepted refugee physicians gained more than they gave, and it is now widely accepted that the presence of refugee physicians from Central Europe has markedly enriched American medicine.

## REFERENCES

1 Remarque EM. *Arch of Triumph*. New York: Appleton-Century Co; 1945.
2 Wikipedia. *Erich Maria Remarque*. Available at: http://en.wikipedia.org/wiki/Erich_Maria_Remarque
3 Remarque, op. cit., p. 97.
4 Kohler ED. *Relicensing Central European Refugee Physicians in the United States, 1933–1945*. Lecture delivered at the Simon Wiesenthal Center, Los Angeles, April 2, 1987. Available at: http://motlc.wiesenthal.com/site/pp.asp?c=gvKVLcMVIuG&b=395145

# CHAPTER 12

# Dr. Yuri Zhivago

## *in Doctor Zhivago*

### by Boris Pasternak[1]

---

### Themes

- How war and revolution disrupt lives and destroy the careers of the survivors
- Collapse of the social structure through revolution and civil war
- A passionate but doomed love affair

---

Boris Leonidovich Pasternak came from an intellectual Jewish family in Moscow. His father was a painter, a professor at the Moscow School of Painting and an illustrator of Tolstoy's works. His mother, Rosa Kaufman, was an accomplished concert pianist. Their home was a magnet for artists, writers and musicians, among them Sergey Rachmaninoff, Alexander Scriabin, Alexander Blok, Andrei Bely and Rainer Maria Rilke. Although first drawn to study music and later philosophy, Pasternak finally settled on literature and started publishing poetry in 1913. In 1921, he produced a volume of poetry named *My Sister Life*, inspired by a passionate love affair he had with a Jewish girl in 1917 while living in the steppe country near Saratov. It, along with the lyric cycle *Rupture*, secured his reputation in Russia as an important poet. In 1922 he married an art student, Eugenia Lurye, and their son, Evgenii, was born the following year.

Originally enthusiastic about the Bolshevik Revolution of 1917, he was soon alienated by the cruelty and brutality of the regime, though it was not until the notorious show trials of the late 1930s that he became thoroughly disillusioned with the oppressive regime. Before that he published a collection of love poems, *Second Birth*, born from his romantic liaison with Zinaida Neigauz, who became his second wife after he divorced Eugenia. During the thirties he tried unsuccessfully to conform his writing style to the socialist realism that was required of all Soviet writers, but he later stopped publishing altogether and made his living translating great foreign writers, among them Shakespeare, Goethe and Rilke.

The last important woman in Pasternak's affection was Olga Ivinskaya, who served as a model for Lara in his brilliant epic novel *Doctor Zhivago*, written in the years 1945 to 1954. The book had no chance of being published in the U.S.S.R. but was smuggled out of the country and appeared in Italy in 1957 to worldwide acclaim and popularity.

In 1958 Pasternak won the Nobel Prize in Literature "for his important achievement in contemporary lyric poetry and in the field of the great Russian epic achievement."[2] The Soviet government, unhappy with his depiction of harsh life under communism, forced him to reject the prize, which he was sadly willing to do because he feared that if he went to Stockholm, the authorities would strip him of his citizenship and force him into exile, something he had struggled to avoid his entire adult life. Pasternak died two years later of lung cancer. It was not until 1988 that the Union of Soviet Writers, from which he had been expelled, posthumously reinstated him, finally allowing publication of *Doctor Zhivago* in his native land. His son Evgenii accepted the Nobel Prize medal on his father's behalf at a ceremony in Stockholm in 1989.

## THE NOVEL

Unlike the author, Yuri Andreievich Zhivago (Yura as a child) is the son of a wastrel and drunkard who abandons his wife and son, squanders the considerable family fortune and finally commits suicide by throwing himself from a moving train. Yura's loving mother dies when he is 10 and he is raised primarily by his mother's brother, Nikolai Nikolaievich Vendeniapin (Uncle Kolia), a cultured man who works for the publisher of the local progressive newspaper in an unnamed provincial town on the Volga, where Yura grows up. Uncle Kolia is the most important influence on his nephew's character and beliefs. Later, while in high school and at the university, Yura lives with the Gromeko family in Moscow. The father, Alexander Alexandrovich, is a chemistry professor. He and his wife, Anna Ivanovna, have a daughter, Antonina (Tonia), who is Yura's age. Although Yura is drawn to poetry and art, he is also fascinated by physics and natural science and decides to become a doctor because he believes that a man should do something socially useful in his practical life. We have glimpses of Yura in the dissecting room studying anatomy and learn later that he is preparing a paper on the nervous elements of the retina for the university's Gold Medal Competition. "His interest in the physiology of sight was in keeping with other sides of his character – his creative gifts and his preoccupation with imagery in art and the logical structure of ideas."[3]

Introduced early in this mélange of characters is Larisa Feodorovna Guishar (Lara), the daughter of a deceased Belgian engineer and a Russianized Frenchwoman, Amalia Karlovna Guishar, whose lover, the lawyer Victor Ippolitovich Komarovsky, is the major villain in this story, suspected by Yura of causing his father's suicide and a shameless seducer of the teenaged Lara.

Yura's marriage to Tonia is preordained by their growing up together and by Anna Invanovna's death-bed wish. As Yura, now grown and called Yuri Andreievich, waits at his hospital for news of the imminent birth of their first child, he thinks about the death of a patient, which he alone of all the attending doctors believed was caused by echinococus of the liver. The autopsy proves him right and his colleagues hail him as a budding diagnostician. The baby, a boy, finally arrives, both mother and child surviving.

Next we see Yuri Andreievich as an army physician at the front, where he is injured during a retreat. Up to this point he and Lara have only seen each other once, at a Christmas party, where the hysterical Lara, still suffering from the shame of her seduction, makes a clumsy attempt to shoot Komarovsky, slightly wounding another man at the same card table instead. Komarovsky manages to squelch the charges against her because he is desperate to keep their relationship a secret. Lara becomes seriously depressed, but later, after she recovers, she marries Pavel Pavlovich Antipov (Pasha), the son of an exiled revolutionary, who has always adored her. They set off for Yuriatin, beyond the Ural Mountains, where they both become teachers and Lara gives birth to their daughter, Katenka. But after Russia's entrance into War World II, Pasha joins the army and for a long time is considered as missing in action, until years later he emerges as a leader of a detachment of Bolshevik partisans fighting the White Army in Siberia.

When Lara, in her search for news about Pasha, arrives at a town behind the front lines, she starts working as a nurse in the hospital ward where Yuri Andreievich is recovering from his wounds and they become reacquainted. Lara knows that she must return to Moscow, collect Katenka and go back to Yuriatin. Meanwhile Yuri reads Tonia's letters, which have caught up with him, and determines that he must go home. News that the Petersburg Garrison has joined the Bolsheviks and that there is street fighting in Petersburg heralds the Revolution. So ends Part One.

But getting home in the midst of revolution, anarchy and civil war is not so easy, and Dr. Yuri Andreievich and Nurse Larisa Antipov must remain and take care of the wounded. The attraction between them is palpable but each is determined to avoid letting it overwhelm them. There is a beautiful description of the spring aromas surrounding the awakening of their love to remind us that Pasternak was essentially a poet.

> All the flowers smelled at once; it was as if the earth, unconscious all day long, were now waking to their fragrance. And from the . . . centuries-old garden, so littered with fallen branches that it was impenetrable, the dusty aroma of old linden trees coming into bloom drifted in a huge wave as tall as a house. . . . Everything was fermenting, growing, rising with the magic yeast of life. The joy of living, like a gentle wind, swept in a broad surge indiscriminately through the fields and towns, through the walls and fences, through wood and flesh. Not to be overwhelmed by this tidal wave, Yuri Andreievich went into the square to listen to the speeches.[4]

When Yuri is back in Moscow with his family – Tonia; her father, Alexander Alexandrovich Gromeko; their son, Sashenka; and Niusha, his nurse – all of them sharing just three rooms of their house, the remaining space assigned to members of the proletariat by the new government, he is working at his old hospital and trying to adjust to the post-revolutionary leveling of society. He not only cares for patients, he is also put in charge of record keeping of patient admissions and deaths, staff earnings, their political consciousness and whether they vote in elections, and tracking inventories of fuel, food and medicines, each in short supply. The bitter winter arrives with its struggle for wood and food. Weakened, Yuri contracts typhus, which is rampant, but slowly recovers. The family decides that it is too dangerous to stay in Moscow and that they should go beyond the Urals, where Tonia's maternal grandfather, old Krueger, owned an estate.

The train trip to the east makes us realize the enormous size of the Soviet Union. It is clear that Pasternak loved the Russian winter from this passage describing how, after an enormous blizzard that shut down all travel, everyone on the train goes to work clearing the track, which takes three days:

> But the sun sparkled on the pure whiteness with a glare that was almost blinding. How cleanly his [Yuri's] shovel cut into its smooth surface! How dry, how iridescent, like diamonds, was each shovelful. He was reminded of the days when, as a child in their yard at home, dressed in a braided hood and a black sheepskin fastened with hooks and eyes sewn into the curly fleece, he cut the dazzling snow into cubes and pyramids and cream puffs and fortresses and the

cities of cave dwellers. Life had had a zest in those far-off days, everything was a feast for the eyes and the stomach. But these three days in the air, too, gave the impression of a feast. And no wonder! At night the workers received loaves of hot fresh bread, which was brought no one knew from where or by whose orders. The bread had a tasty crisp crust, shiny on top, cracked at the side, and with bits of charcoal baked into it underneath.[5]

They settle into the abandoned Krueger house and, following Tolstoy's example, they live off the land. Yuri doesn't practice medicine; he writes poems and records his observations about the meaning of the Revolution and the changes it has wrought. He goes periodically to Yuriatin on horseback to do research at the library. And there he rediscovers Lara. This time there is no inhibition; they become lovers. Yuri is awash in guilt because he also loves his wife, now pregnant with their second child, but in a different way – they are friends and they admire and respect each other. But with Lara this is unrestrained passion that cannot be suppressed.

Riding home from Yuriatin after a rendezvous with Lara late one afternoon, he is accosted by Red Army partisans, who conscript him into their unit on the spot because their doctor has been killed, carrying him off without allowing him to contact his family. Yuri becomes a prisoner-doctor, treating the wounded, the many cases of typhus and dysentery and one soldier, utterly devoted to the revolution, whom his superiors value but describe as a "mental case," apparently suffering from what we now call post-traumatic stress disorder. Yuri complains to his superiors that he does not have sufficient transport for the wounded when the unit moves, and that he must rely on the few medicines they have – quinine, Glauber's salts, iodine. He is appalled that the destruction of the vodka still, ordered to cut down drunkenness among the soldiers, means there is no alcohol, which he needs to dissolve the iodine crystals so that they are usable in surgery and for dressings. The still is reconstructed and the brewers are told to make alcohol for medical purposes only, but soon drunkenness reappears.

Meanwhile in the wilds of Siberia Yuri comes across a famous partisan leader called Strelnikov, Lara's missing husband Pasha, who recognizes that Lara loves someone else. Yuri worries about Tonia and how she will manage her confinement and about his son, who is growing up without a father. But it is Lara he dreams of.

How he loved her! How beautiful she was! In exactly the way he had always thought and dreamed and wanted! Yet what was it that made her so lovely? Was it something that could be named and analyzed? No, a thousand times no!

She was lovely by virtue of the matchlessly simple and swift line that the Creator had, at a single stroke, drawn all around her, and in this divine form she had been handed over, like a child tightly wrapped in a sheet after its bath, into the keeping of his soul.[6]

Finally, desperate, he escapes from the partisans and, after weeks of walking, manages to get to Yuriatin, debilitated, exhausted and a shadow of his former self. Lara nurses him back to health, telling him that she helped Tonia with her delivery, that he has a daughter and that the family has gone back to Moscow. Their reunion is joyful, sensuous, compelling. Although they both sense they have not much time together – Yuri must try to rejoin his family, Lara and Katenka are in danger because her husband Strelnikov has enemies in high places – they nonetheless go off to the Krueger farm for whatever tiny scrap of time they can capture. It is here that Pasternak has written a love story for the ages, a story of lovers doomed to part forever. Lara must seek safety in the Far East and Yuri must return to his family in Moscow.

Once there he finds that Tonia, her father and the children have been forced to emigrate and are living in Paris. By now it is 1922, the civil war is over, the Bolsheviks are in full control and re-education has become a way of life for those whom the regime doesn't trust. While waiting for a job to open up, Yuri writes poetry. But he has only a few years to live and, though not yet 40, he believes he suffers from sclerosis of the heart, which he describes to his friends as follows:

"Microscopic forms of cardiac hemorrhages have become very frequent in recent years. They are not always fatal. Some people get over them. It's a typical modern disease. I think its causes are of a moral order. The great majority of us are required to live a life of constant, systematic duplicity. Your health is bound to be affected if, day after day, you say the opposite of what you feel, if you grovel before what you dislike and rejoice at what brings you nothing but misfortune. Our nervous system isn't just a fiction, it's part of our physical body, and our soul exists in space and is inside us, like the teeth in our mouth. It can't be forever violated with impunity. I found it painful to listen to you, Innokentii, when you told us how you were re-educated and became mature in jail. It was like listening to a horse describe how it broke itself in."[7]

Thus Yuri Andreievich comes to see all that has happened in Russia for what it really is, a new form of tyranny and despotism, more authoritarian and cruel than the old Tsarist regime. How this milieu actually contributed to the death of Dr. Zhivago is not explained. The description of his heart ailment, with thinning heart walls ready to burst and minuscule hemorrhages in the heart, makes little sense from a medical perspective. Pasternak might have lacked a medical consultant or simply used his *licentia poetica*. Indeed, it can be argued that Zhivago was more a poet and lover than a doctor and in another age most likely would have given up medicine for writing, as did Anton Chekhov and A.J. Cronin. This is borne out by the collection of Yuri's poems at the end of the novel and the following stanza from a poem called 'Parting':

> When one no longer sees the day
> Because of hoarfrost on the panes
> The hopelessness of grief redoubles
> Its likeness to the sea's vast desert.[8]

Pasternak makes his hero a doctor not to view the medical scene in Russia but to stress Yuri's desire to be useful to society and to allow him to witness at close range the tragedies of the civil war and to be in a place where he meets a nurse with whom he is destined to fall in love.

To read this novel in a good translation is to enjoy a swift narrative, to follow an intricate plot played out on the stage of the immense Russian landscape, to shudder at the horrors of the bloody revolution and the suffering of its victims and to feel the pain of the lovers' separation, a theme that wars and revolutions have nourished in the imagination of writers and composers since time immemorial. The reader lured by the word Doctor in the title will not find much doctoring, but will be rewarded by the beauty of the prose and the depth of human emotions contained in this literary gem, justly honored by the Nobel award that the author was forced to decline. In this he is joined by Solzhenitsyn, who was barred from attending his award ceremony in 1970. Declining the Nobel Prize was rare, although earlier, in 1901, Leo Tolstoy told the Nobel Committee that was preparing to give him the award that he was refusing any further prizes. Of Western writers, Jean-Paul Sartre declined the official honor of the Nobel Prize in 1964 and a Swedish poet, E.A. Karfeldt, refused the award in 1918 but accepted it in 1931.[9]

## REFERENCES

1 Pasternak B (1945–56). *Doctor Zhivago*. Translation by Max Hayward and Manya Harari. New York: Pantheon Books; 1958.
2 Nobelprize.org. *The Nobel Prize in Literature 1958*. Available at: http://nobelprize.org/nobel_prizes/literature/laureates/1958/
3 Pasternak, op. cit., p. 65.
4 Ibid., p. 79.

5 Ibid., pp. 140–1.
6 Ibid., pp. 229–30.
7 Ibid., p. 367.
8 Ibid., p. 543.
9 Wikipedia. Nobel Prize in Literature. Available at: http://en.wikipedia.org/wiki/Nobel_Prize_in_Literature

## PART FOUR

# Novel psychiatrists

# CHAPTER 13

# Dr. Dick Diver

## in *Tender is the Night*
### by F. Scott Fitzgerald[1]

---

### Themes

- ■ Physician's idle life leads to decadence and torpor
- ■ Negative transference, or "Never Marry a Patient"
- ■ The hourglass of vitality

---

The hero of this novel is a physician who happens to be a psychiatrist, but this occupation serves only to explain his involvement with a patient, whom he marries and who will change the path of his life. The author's treatment of psychiatry and a few sketches of psychiatric patients lack not only depth but even a rudimentary understanding of the various psychiatric illnesses and the professional activities of a psychiatrist. In a sense, however, Dick Diver's inability to control his own downward slide in life is ironical for he is a doctor who is supposed to help people change even as he cannot change himself. Though the book cannot be taken as a reflection on medicine and psychiatry, it remains a major masterpiece of American literature during the period between the two world wars.

F. Scott Fitzgerald (1896–1940), named for his famous relative Francis Scott Keys, is so identified with the Jazz Age that some early criticism did not take him seriously as a writer, though later more thoughtful analysis by the literary world recognized his enormous gifts and established his reputation as a great American writer. He was born in St. Paul, Minnesota to an upper-middle-class Irish Catholic family in 1896, and he was educated at St. Paul Academy, the Neuman School in Hackensack, N.J. and Princeton University, where he wrote for the Princeton Triangle Club. He dropped out of college in 1917 to enlist in the army and was stationed at Camp Sheridan, where he fell in love with Zelda Sayre, a young socialite in Montgomery, Alabama, who was the daughter of an Alabama Supreme Court Judge. His first novel, *This Side of Paradise*, about the post-war flappers, was published in 1920 and became a huge success. Scott and Zelda were married in St. Patrick's Cathedral that year, and their only child, Frances Scott Fitzgerald, was born in 1921. In 1925 Fitzgerald published *The Great Gatsby*, thought by many critics to be the finest American novel ever written.

Much of Fitzgerald's writing was autobiographical. His father lost his prestigious job with Procter and Gamble when Scott was 12, so he knew about financial loss, and money – its absence or presence in large amounts – played a central role in his life and writing. His early success launched the Fitzgeralds on an opulent lifestyle that none of his later book royalties could support, so he supplemented his income by writing short stories for popular magazines. He was an alcoholic, as are several of his heroes, and alcohol is prominently involved in the partying lifestyle of the twenties portrayed in his fiction. He had a hard time capturing Zelda, who once broke off their engagement until he impressed her with the big splash created by his first novel, and the male wooing of the golden girl figures prominently in his fiction. His wife's intense and flamboyant personality was the model for many of his heroines and, after she was diagnosed with schizophrenia in 1930, for Nicole Diver in *Tender is the Night*.

**THE STORY**

Dr. Richard Diver arrives in Zurich in 1917, at the age of 26, to continue his scientific work in a psychiatric hospital. A handsome, intelligent and charming young man, Diver is an Oxford Rhodes Scholar, a graduate of Johns Hopkins and a student of Freud in Vienna. His father is a physician and one of his ancestors was a governor of North Carolina. His colleagues in Vienna call him "Lucky Dick." He attracts the almost instant affection of men and women crossing his path, as he charms them with his graceful manners and outstanding vitality, exhibiting his extraordinary virtuosity with people. Nicole, Dick's wife, feels that he has the power of arousing a fascinating and uncritical love in everybody he might come across.

Nicole is a very beautiful, fragile, capricious, immensely rich young American patient at the institution where Dick pursues his studies and gathers material for his scientific writing. The nature of her psychiatric illness never becomes entirely clear. She is an incest victim and is listed as a schizophrenic, but after a stormy childhood and adolescence she is much improved, even, perhaps, nearly recovered and acting more like a spoiled brat than a mental patient. (Our psychoanalytical reviewer finds it surprising that, with such excellent training, Dr. Diver ignored the boundary problem created by becoming emotionally involved with a patient – an absolute no-no in psychiatry – which would lead inevitably to narcissistic conflict and mutual hatred. Furthermore she believes that Nicole is not schizophrenic at all but rather has a poorly integrated personality.)

Nicole is immediately attracted to Dick and, after the U.S. enters the war, finds him even more alluring in his captain's uniform. He completely captivates Nicole; his absence only adds fuel to her romantic fantasies and she pursues him with letters and titillates him with flattery and adulation. Nicole's obsession with Dick apparently gives her a therapeutic boost; at least this is what her physicians believe, telling Dick he has accomplished an unusually effective and fortuitous transference. The problem of coping with a seductive patient is very much publicized today but might not have been an important issue in the 1920s. Dick's influence on Nicole's illness and her youth, beauty and romantic love easily dissolve whatever might have constituted sensible and ethical resistance. They are both drawn indelibly to each other, perhaps more physically than intellectually. But the strongest bond seems to be the patient–doctor relationship, which lasts throughout their courtship, marriage and the raising of their children. During this period Nicole has frequent relapses, which play havoc with her ability to cope. She is severely depressed after childbirth, and Dick must summon the maximum of professional competence, patience and detachment to be a successful therapist.

When Nicole is not suffering from a delusional paranoia or depression, she is a lovely creature and a good companion. When she is ill, she is in an agony of despair. It seems Fitzgerald was not much concerned with drawing a consistent pattern of a definite psychiatric entity. Instead he mixes features of anxiety, hysteria, manic depressive illness, schizophrenia and personality disorder. However, mental patients often do have more than one illness. Fitzgerald lived with this; his wife, Zelda, was the model for Nicole. Dick's role appears mostly to be to protect and support Nicole during her relapses into psychotic behavior.

They marry in 1919 and their marriage dissolves in 1930. Toward the end, Nicole becomes stronger and more balanced, while Dick gradually disintegrates, a victim of alcoholism and a purposeless existence. Shortly before they part, she tells him that he used to create things and now he seems to want to smash them. She asks what he gets out of this behavior. The answer is: "knowing you are stronger every day, knowing that your illness follows the law of diminishing returns."[2] Now it should be Nicole's turn to protect and support him but she has no intention of helping Dick, of trying to bring him out of his inertia and save him from alcoholism. That role reversal does not take place, only the switch in the role of victim occurs. Nicole cannot tell him what he should or should not do, even though she feels sorry for him – sorry not as a lover or friend but as someone who was once mentally afflicted. There is no memory of his love, devotion and dedication to curing her. Dick has ceased to exercise control, he has become useless and superfluous, and Nicole walks away with a younger and stronger lover, taking their children and all her material wealth.

## Dr. Diver's practice of psychiatry

About seven years after Dick and Nicole marry, seven years of a rich and idle existence on the Riviera and in Paris, Nicole's money is invested in a partnership in one of the most modern and best-equipped psychiatric clinics in Europe, located south of Zurich on the Zugersee. There is a scattering of elegant cottages tastefully decorated by Nicole. We learn little about Dick's medical practice except for his warmth, sincerity and empathy. His rounds resemble a sort of laying on of hands for the suffering, mostly unfortunate rich inmates for whom medicine probably cannot do much because they seem more like physically decaying wrecks than victims of psychiatric illnesses. From the few sketchy episodes of Dick's ministering, it does not seem clear whether the author has a notion of the line which separates the physician psychiatrist from the psychologist or lay therapist.

## Dick's scientific writing

Dick returned to Zurich after the war with a set of notes arranged into a book called *A Psychology for Psychiatrists*. The content is never revealed and we do not know why Dick is qualified to write a textbook on such an improbable if not meaningless subject, and what might have been the purpose and message of the treatise. The book was apparently published in German, and as soon as this occurred he started planning a new work entitled *An attempt at a uniform and pragmatic classification of the neurosis and psychoses based on an examination of fifteen hundred Pre-Kraepelin and Post-Kraepelin cases as they would be diagnosed in the terminology of the different contemporary schools – together with a chronology of such subdivisions of opinion as have arisen independently.*[3] This absurd title implies some gigantic opus that would look monumental in German, which pleases Dick. But even the word naive would not be fitting for this kind of a grandiose and megalomaniac undertaking. To complete 1500 case histories would require the lifetime of not one but 10 or 20 psychiatrists. Such an idea could not have entered the mind of a young, relatively inexperienced, charming playboy, as Dick was described at that point in his life.

During the next six or seven years Dick enjoys the life of a rich expatriate in the company of mostly sterile writers and artists, partying, traveling and keeping an eye on Nicole's emotional balance. Yet during his spare time he is preparing the second volume of *The Psychology for Psychiatrists*, which has reached in German the absurd number of 50 editions. Here the author decides to terminate Dick's creativity by revealing that, like so many men he has seen, he had only one or two good ideas and that his first book contained the essence of everything that he would think or know in the future. In this transition from a successful medical authority to a totally washed-out intellectual wreck, Fitzgerald does not bother to explain this loss of talent, drive and expertise. It seems that he is concerned with the sterility of an artist and does not bother to distinguish the writing of fiction from scientific writing, which is not a product of inspiration but of research and experimental or practical experiences, commodities not readily acquired in Dick's situation. Indeed, had they been present they would not be inexplicably lost in a moment of self-searching that brings on a flash of insight.

### Dick's corruption by the rich and idle life

Although Dick scrupulously avoids using Nicole's money for himself, her wealth permeates his lifestyle and affects his moves. It is Nicole who decides that they must leave Zurich to live near a warm beach where they can be young and beautiful and brown together. He seems very content with his life on the Riviera and in Paris among the wealthy and glamorous, a life of partying, shopping, bar hopping and flirting. At the time he confesses that although he has wasted nine years teaching the rich the ABCs of human decency, he nonetheless still believes he has many unplayed trumps in his hand. There is no clear road to recovery in sight, however, and the statement lacks credibility.

### Dick's self-destruction

This is not the result of a plausibly developed process. He seems to tire of Nicole's fits of irrational behavior, travels alone, has a fleeting and unsatisfactory affair with a much younger American movie actress, Rosemary, rejects her, becomes absurdly drunk, enters a bar-room brawl, punches a policeman and is savagely beaten and jailed in Rome. He continues drinking after his return to the clinic, averaging half a pint of alcohol a day, too much for his system to burn up. He is free to leave the clinic and travels aimlessly for another year through Europe with his family, while a seemingly incurable alcoholic. After Nicole leaves him, he returns to the United States, where he at first opens an office to practice medicine in Buffalo, apparently without success, then moves to a smaller town. There is a hint of a scandal and a lawsuit, and finally he fades away from the scene with the vague allusion of total disintegration. There is no longer any communication with Nicole.

Dick Diver is hardly a model of a physician or a psychiatrist. The profession is accidental to the intended theme of a talented, successful young man corrupted by the purposeless life amid the rich and idle, culminating in self-destruction by alcohol. This is a highly autobiographical novel mirroring Fitzgerald's own decline – in his case victim of premature fame, a mentally ill wife and alcoholism. However, while the novel flows like sand in an hourglass, the sand being Dick's strength and vitality flowing into Nicole and emptying him of all energy and emotion, in Fitzgerald's own life Zelda did not grow stronger as his life was falling apart; if she was a vampire drinking his blood, she failed to prosper from it.

## REFERENCES

1 Fitzgerald FS (1934). *Tender is the Night*. New York; Scribner; 1942.
2 Ibid., p. 273.
3 Ibid., p. 140.

## CHAPTER 14

# Dr. Howard Berger

## in *Ordinary People*

### by Judith Guest[1]

---

### Themes

- Teenage depression
- Attempted suicide in adolescents
- Sympathetic therapist

---

This first novel was turned down by many publishers, but when it appeared it became an instant best-seller, probably because of two timely themes – first, a reminder that a sudden catastrophic accident can shatter the lives of "ordinary people" in more than one way; second, that either attempted or successful suicide in the teen population is particularly tragic and devastating to family and friends. The book's success started Judith Guest, a teacher and the mother of three sons, on her career as a novelist. Begun as a short story, *Ordinary People* grew into a novel after she became intrigued by the prevalence of teenage depression.

In this case disaster strikes the upper-middle-class Jarrett family of Chicago when one of their sons drowns in a boating accident. The two boys are best friends and overachievers both scholastically and in athletics. The victim, Buck, has the more outgoing personality; his younger brother, Conrad, is more withdrawn. The drawback of the novel is that we know little of the family dynamics before the tragedy, which may be important in understanding the parents' reactions to the tragedy. However, the title "Ordinary" indicates the lack of deep fissures in their lives. The accident tears apart the marriage of the parents, who cannot find common ground in coping with the loss of their older son and the ensuing depression and attempted suicide of his younger brother. The latter is the main theme of the novel.

In the 1970s, when the action of the novel takes place, depression and suicide among teenagers was only beginning to emerge as a serious public health problem. But depression and suicide are now of epidemic proportions in America.[2] Suicide rates have tripled since 1970, making it, after auto accidents, the second leading cause of death among 15 to 24 year olds.[3] In one recent survey of high school students, 20% said they had thought about killing themselves and about 8% said they had tried at least once.[4] In the United States male adolescents commit suicide at a rate that is five times greater than that of female adolescents.[5]

Our interest in this novel focuses on Howard Berger, M.D., the psychiatrist who treats Conrad Jarrett, the 17-year-old hero of the story, a youngster deeply depressed since his brother drowned when their sailboat overturned during an unexpected storm on Lake Michigan. As the novel opens, Conrad, who is an intelligent and talented upper-class student, has been released from the mental hospital where he spent eight months after an attempted suicide. Berger is the follow-up doctor, probably 30 to 40 years old, practicing in a somewhat dilapidated section of Chicago. Dr. Berger is most unprofessionally attired in a crumpled sweater, sitting sometimes with his legs folded under him, sometimes hunched up like a crafty monkey. He has sharp stinging blue eyes, which he casts on his patients like a beam, and a darkened face upon which grows tufts of dark crinkly hair. He drinks coffee incessantly, munches sweet rolls and transacts his business to provide a semblance of informality and to relax Conrad and help him open up.

Conrad is not initially charmed by Dr. Berger, as he has acquired a deep suspicion of this breed of doctors and their put-on eccentricities that he witnessed in the hospital. But gradually you see Berger's common sense and gently kidding approach to the teenager working to help rid him of the guilt he carries about surviving when his brother did not, the insecurities that make integrating back into his high school life difficult, and the problem he has with his mother, who is unable to show love.

One of Berger's great strengths is his availability in a pinch. When Conrad reads in the local paper that a girl he befriended at the hospital, who seemed to be fine in their one post-hospital get-together, has committed suicide, he goes to pieces and calls Berger at home at 6 a.m. after a sleepless and tortured night. The doctor sees him at once. The scene that follows is the best in the novel, as Berger dissolves Conrad's self-blame by recreating step by step the details of the boating accident, forcing Conrad to admit that Buck was both physically stronger than he and a better swimmer. Finally, he asks Conrad what he thinks he could have done to keep Buck from drowning. He demonstrates that Conrad's pain is related to his trying to be Buck for the sake of his parents and grandparents, but that he will never succeed, that what he needs to do is to be himself. Gradually released from his insecure and self-hating mood, Conrad becomes increasingly stronger. He gets up the nerve to ask a girl he likes for a date and doesn't run away when their relationship deepens. He also repairs the break with his best friend that had occurred after Buck's death. The patient and doctor become friends, and we know that Conrad is going to make it back to the real world in a relatively healthy condition.

His parents are less lucky. His mother's problem of being unable to show Conrad love, possibly because she never wants to be hurt again the way she was when Buck died, seems like highly improbable behavior, but it does lead to her withdrawal and the end of the marriage. Thus the novel avoids an unrealistically upbeat ending and is rather like real life, where things don't always turn out the way you want them to.

Dr. Berger does not fit the stereotype of an intelligent and erudite analyst probing the mind of a patient stretched on his office couch, but one prefers to believe that he is a real flesh-and-blood physician available when a patient is in emotional turmoil – someone who understands human psychology and is willing to apply this knowledge to form strong bonds with his patients, with affection and the generous gift of his time. We don't know whether the author encountered someone like Dr. Berger in real life or conceived him in her imagination as the ideal omniscient and compassionate mind healer, but the psychiatric profession should always welcome doctors with these attributes.

## REFERENCES

1 Guest J. *Ordinary People*. New York: Ballantine Books, acquired by Random House; 1976.
2 Wilkinson, W. The Great Depression: is an epidemic of depressive disorder really sweeping America? *Reason Online*. December 2007. Available at: www.reason.com/news/show/123024.html
3 Centers for Disease Control and Prevention. *Suicide Fact Sheet*. 30 March 2006. Available at: www.cdc.gov/ (accessed 2 May 2006).
4 Cartuso, K. *How Common is it for High School Students to Consider Suicide?* Available at: www.suicide.org/high-school-students-suicide.html
5 National Youth Violence Prevention Resource Center. *Youth Suicide Fact Sheet*. Available at: www.safeyouth.org/scripts/facts/suicide.asp. 1 January 2005.

# CHAPTER 15

# Dr. Johanna Von Haller

## in *The Manticore*

### by Robertson Davies[1]

---

### Themes

- ◼ Jungian analysis and the archetypes
- ◼ Continuation of *Deptford* saga

---

Robertson Davies was a Canadian novelist, playwright, critic and journalist and was professor at Upper Canada College in Toronto, Queens University in Kingston, Ontario, and Balliol College, Oxford. As an aspiring actor he played small roles at the Old Vic Repertory Company in London. Back home in Toronto he worked at various newspapers, writing essays and literary criticism. He wrote a prize-winning one-act play but found his greatest success in fiction. He is the author of 11 major novels, among them *The Cunning Man*, discussed in the next chapter. Always fascinated by myth and magic, two themes that appear in several of his novels, he wrote *The Manticore* to exemplify the method of psyche exploration developed by the Swiss psychiatrist Carl Jung (1875–1961), whose work fascinated him. In fact, the novel is cast as a Jungian analysis.[2]

Carl Jung's theory claims that the psyche has three parts – the ego, or consciousness; the personal unconscious, or memories both readily accessible and suppressed; and the collective unconscious, or our experiences as a species, our "psychic inheritance." Jung called the contents of the collective unconscious "archetypes," which form a dynamic substratum common to all humanity and from which each individual builds his or her own experiences, developing a unique array of psychological characteristics. Jung described archetypal events, such as birth, death, separation from parents and marriage, as well as archetypal figures, such as mother, father, child, God, trickster, hero and wise old man. He also proposed the existence of the Self, the anima, the animus and the shadow as psychological structures having an archetypal nature.[3]

## THE STORY

David Staunton, a wealthy and successful 42-year-old Canadian lawyer, is, at the start of this novel, a vastly unhappy man, depressed, alcoholic, sharp-tongued even to people he cares for, uninterested in sex, loaded with self-hatred and frightened that he is going mad. His father, Boy Staunton, a highly successful industrialist, philanthropist and politician, has just died under mysterious circumstances, driving his car at high speed into a lake. When his body was retrieved, he had a stone in his mouth. Whether this was suicide or accident is not clear, but it is this tragedy that has brought David to Zurich, where he seeks therapeutic help through Jungian analysis. He describes his pain as "That heavy axe that seems always to be chopping away at the roots of my being."[4]

In the novel *Fifth Business*, part of *The Deptford Trilogy* and preceding *The Manticore*, the young Boy Staunton throws a snowball containing a stone at his friend, Dunstan Ramsey, but Ramsey ducks and the snowball strikes the head of a passerby, the pregnant wife of Reverend Dempster. This event will affect the lives of three boys, whose stories are told in the trilogy, Boy Staunton, Dunstan Ramsey and the newborn Paul Dempster.

After his initial interview with the director of the Jung Institute, but before he ever meets his therapist, David has a dream about leaving a college campus where he feels comfortable and safe, though he experiences the terrain outside as strange and frightening. There he meets an unknown woman who is trying to tell him something important that he cannot or will not understand. After he meets his therapist, Dr. Johanna Von Haller, and recovers from the shock that he is to be treated by a woman, he understands that the woman in the dream represents his therapist, and that he is ambivalent at best, and resistant at worst, to whatever she will tell him in the course of his treatment. This is not unusual among patients starting therapy, who often feel simultaneously positive and negative about their decision to enter analysis. In David's case, this reaction is aggravated by the fact that he has not admired the psychiatrists he has seen testifying as witnesses in court.

Johanna Von Haller is a beautiful and elegant woman about Staunton's own age, who is happily married though aware that many men fall in love with her during their analyses. She is careful never to allow her professional relationships to extend to social or personal contact with her patients. She is almost a romanticized figure of an analyst, endowed with empathy, wisdom and a skilled methodology of unearthing the unconscious and guiding her patients from confusion to coherence.

Despite his initial ambivalence, David comes to see her as "altogether a person to inspire confidence;"[5] this is important because it allows him to accept, after numerous battles, her explanations of his psychic state and her assertion that the doctor–patient relationship must be one of mutual respect. She insists that it is not unusual for patients to have important and revealing dreams before meeting their doctors and that "perhaps despite coming to the Institute for help, he doesn't really want to hear what she has to say."[6]

Early in David's therapy, Von Haller picks up on his excessive drinking, a bottle of whiskey a day, and warns him that this will adversely affect his health. She advises him to leave his luxury hotel and find a pension without a bar, which his upper-class world-view finds distasteful, although later he follows her advice. She explains to David, who is anxious to know what his therapy will entail, that she will use many techniques to start the stream of recollection flowing and to bring out clues about what is important to him. In turn, she wants to know what he expects from therapy – a cure for his drinking? To gain needed maturity? Better relations with his family members?

Later in her analysis, Dr. Von Haller finds nothing wrong with his thinking and reasoning but exposes great defects in his emotional life and underlying feelings and a severe imbalance between his relation to his father and his mother. He is not, however, psychotic, she says, but he is in an unsatisfactory state of mind that he wants to resolve. Staunton thinks describing his emotional state merely as an unsatisfactory state of mind is far too mild a description of his suffering.

David has spent his life admiring, even adoring, his father, while insisting on making his own way without Boy Staunton's financial help, which he does successfully, as he is bright, well trained and an excellent advocate. Although he longs for paternal approbation, he refuses to do the one thing his father wants – marry and have a family to carry on the Staunton name. David's aversion to marriage and women in general stems from the way he was introduced to sex at age 17 – an arranged candlelight dinner with one of his father's mistresses, which has left a permanent emotional scar. This was aggravated by the enforced separation from the girl he really loved, Judy Wolff, whose father shipped her off to boarding school in Europe because the religious and class differences between their families would make their eventual marriage impossible. Boy Staunton inflicts another punishment from beyond the grave, leaving David nothing in his will except the family foundation to manage and, twisting the knife of his final displeasure a little deeper, financial provision for any children he might have.

His mother is another story – a great beauty from a poor family in their home town of Deptford, who, unable to become a credible socialite, could not live up to her husband's expectations. David feels genuine love for her but also pity for her dependent character and frequent illnesses. Then there is his lively and manipulative sister, Caroline, and his long-time nurse and later the family housekeeper, Netty, who has been a strong influence in his life.

As David tells the story of his childhood and adolescence – his history of winters in Toronto with his parents and summers in Deptford with his grandparents – he elaborates on his colorful Grandfather Staunton, who was a physician by profession but was mainly occupied by raising sugar beets on a large scale and manufacturing them into raw sugar. Grandpa owned land, factories and railroads, making the Stauntons the richest family in town. He was a tall, broad, fat gentleman with a big stomach and a large, strawberry-red nose. He had qualified as a physician in 1887, but before that he had been an apprentice to Dr. Gamsby, the first doctor ever to come to Deptford, and he still possessed Gamsby's professional equipment, which lay in disorder and neglect in a couple of glass-fronted cases in his office. He loved to tell stories about how some of these gadgets had been employed in the old days. His favorite was the scarifier, which was used on patients who complained they couldn't move because of rheumatism. The doctor placed it against the stiff area and pressed a button that released 12 sharp blade points an eighth of an inch long, which caused the sufferer not to just move but to leap. This story always produced a big laugh from Grandfather Staunton. He also fought a major campaign against constipation, which the local farmers, dreading their freezing privies in winter, encouraged by developing abnormal powers of retention. Grandfather Staunton brought the constipation wars home, dosing young David with cascara sagrada at night and Epsom salts in the morning.

But David suffers much more searing recollections than his grandfather's outdated medical practices – rage at his father for arranging his sexual introduction and for being a philanderer; Caroline's insistence that he is actually the child of Dunstan Ramsey, whom she believes was their mother's lover; Caroline's suspicion that their mother either committed suicide by opening the window and letting in the chill that killed her when she was already ill or, worse, that Netty was the culprit because of her rapturous love for their father; David's hatred of Netty's beloved brother, Matey, whom he calls "a loathsome little squirt."[7] Caroline's suppositions reflect her own neurotic imagination, since it is clear that Dunstan Ramsey is not David's father, though her suspicions about Netty as her mother's murderer may or may not be valid.

Von Haller introduces the Jungian archetypes as a way of helping David to untangle his tortured emotional life. First there is the Shadow, that negative and rarely admitted side of oneself. Slowly David comes to see that his deep dislike of Matey stems from seeing in Matey's character the things he dislikes about himself and that he has made Matey his scapegoat. We are not trying to banish the Shadow, explains Dr. Von Haller, only to understand it. Her point, an important one, is that David must know what he is doing subconsciously in order to examine his dark corner effectively and overcome it. She says that as David learns to recognize how he projects the parts of himself that he dislikes onto others, he'll be able to control them; he'll be stronger, more independent and have more mental energy.

Late in the novel David has accepted and internalized this concept:

> Dr. Johanna has freed me from many a bogey, but she has also sharpened my already razorlike ethical sense. In her terms I have always projected the Shadow onto Matey; I have seen him as the worst of myself. I have been a heel in too many ways to count ... worst of all miserable to Father about things where he was vulnerable and I was strong. The account is long and disgusting. I have accepted all that; it is part of what I am and unless I know it, grasp it, and acknowledge it as my own, there can be no freedom for me and no hope of being a less miserable stinker in the future.[8]

There are other archetypes – the Anima, the feminine side of himself, where David is rich because of the women in his life – his mother, Caroline, Netty, Judy, even Denyse, his hated stepmother, whom Von Haller calls an unfriendly anima. Finally, there is the archetype Persona, which is himself, and the Magus or Wizard or Guru, a role she believes Dunstan Ramsey, the boy who ducked the ominous stone and grew up to be one of David's college professors, has played in his life.

By this time, David admits to himself and to Von Haller that he is in love with her, a very familiar occurrence in analysis. And finally we get to the manticore in the following dream:

David is in an underground passage that feels and appears to be Roman. Etched on the left wall is a life-size picture of Dr. Von Haller, dressed as a sibyl (prophet) in a white robe with a blue mantle, smiling a very beautiful calm smile, and holding on a chain a lion who has David's face. The lion's tail is spiked. Von Haller practically claps her hands in joy as she explains that the lion is actually a manticore, a creature with a lion's body, a man's face and a sting in his tail. When David wonders how he could possibly dream of something he has never heard of, Von Haller says it is common because "great myths are not invented stories but objectifications of images and situations that lie very deep in the human spirit."[9]

David interprets the dream to mean he is in her power on a very short leash. Von Haller questions whether she really is the woman in the dream, though she says that this woman is someone he loves and asks if this woman also loves him. He says yes, or at least that she is someone who cares about him. Next she asks why he is a manticore. David doesn't know but says he supposes the manticore represents his baser side, but not entirely base because a lion is a noble creature, and not entirely animal because it has a human face. She returns to where David is weak and asks, "So might not your undeveloped feeling turn up in a dream as a noble creature, but possibly dangerous and only human in part?"[10] In short, it is a likeness of himself when in court. Then she leads him to see that the sibyl in the dream is his Anima, his feminine side.

By this time David has been in Zurich for a year; the Christmas holidays loom as Von Haller sums up the positive effects of the analysis – his drinking is now moderate, his general health better, his sleep untroubled, and he's a much more pleasant person to deal with. The question now is whether to continue and finish the work, which allows patients to deepen their understanding of themselves and have greater control of their abilities. She asks him to consider this and come to a decision over the Christmas holidays.

David goes to St. Gall, where he meets Dunstan Ramsey by a wild coincidence. Ramsey is with an ugly woman named Doctor Liselotte Naegeli (Liesl). We don't know what kind of a doctor she is. They invite him to her castle, Sorgenfrei, for Christmas. The upshot of this encounter is that David must choose between staying and working with Dr. Von Haller or taking Liesl's advice and doing his own self-analysis, with an implication that more may be forthcoming from Liesl than the promised friendship. David is now a relatively happy man, so it doesn't really matter what he decides and we do not find out.

We have to admit that reading *The Manticore* in isolation may be puzzling, but the novel fits well in the context of the entire trilogy, which we strongly recommend. In itself it is an interesting book because the writing is excellent and the story of unearthing "archetypes" intriguing. The length and cost of analysis and the methods of interrogation about past events and patients' dreams by the Jungians resemble Freudian analysis, though perhaps with a lesser exploration of the libido and greater exploration of personality development in terms of universal archetypes.

## DIVERSE PSYCHIATRIC PRACTICES

The three novels we have discussed featuring practicing psychiatrists have little in common regarding the approach used in treating disturbed patients. Psychoanalytic treatment by Dr. Von Haller is a very long process, which only a small fraction of wealthy and intelligent clients can afford. It is aimed at eliminating neurosis and altering patients' self-image to achieve a permanent cure.

Dr. Berger's goal is more limited and the treatment course is shorter. It is a commonsense improvisation aimed at reinterpreting bothersome events, absolving the patient of self-incrimination and restoring mental equilibrium. This is a more practical and affordable approach than psychoanalytic dissection but, if treatment is not continued, the goal is limited to alleviating a single crisis.

Dr. Diver's role (*see* Chapter 13) is palliation of intermittent psychotic relapses of his wife, but her psychiatric diagnosis is not defined, and he commits a grave error by marrying a patient and then treating his own wife. As mentioned earlier, Scott Fitzgerald had no real understanding of the practice of psychiatry; his aim was to portray a certain segment of society at a particular time in history, a time he knew well from personal experience.

## REFERENCES

1 Davies R (1972). *The Manticore.* Toronto: Penguin Group (Canada); 2005.
2 Encylopedia.com. *Robertson Davies. The Columbia Encyclopedia.* 6th ed. 2008. Available at: www.encyclopedia.com/doc/1E1-DaviesR.html; Jordan K. *A Biography of Robertson Davies: the creator of* The Deptford Trilogy. September 25, 2007. Available at: http://modern-canadian-history.suite101.com/article.cfm/robertson_davies; Wikipedia. *Robertson Davies.* Available at: http://en.wikipedia.org/wiki/Robertson_Davies
3 Boeree CG, M.D. *Carl Jung.* Available at: http://webspace.ship.edu/cgboer/jung.html
4 Davies, op. cit., pp. 46–7.
5 Ibid., p. 9.
6 Ibid., p. 16.
7 Ibid., p. 112.
8 Ibid., p. 219.
9 Ibid., p. 145.
10 Ibid., p. 147.

# CHAPTER 16

# Dr. Jonathan Hullah

in *The Cunning Man*

by Robertson Davies[1]

---

### Themes

- Medicine is part art and part science
- Psychosomatic medicine
- The advantages of independent wealth in the practice of medicine

---

Although most of Robertson Davies' novels are arranged as trilogies, with material drawn from two diverse sources – the examination of Canadian society and his in-depth knowledge of Western civilization, encompassing literature, history, music, art, philosophy and psychology – *The Cunning Man* stands alone, perhaps because it is his final novel. Characterized by his usual exquisite prose, interesting characters, mostly from the educated echelon of society, and an interesting plot, it provides a gratifying reading experience. The critic of the *Boston Sunday Globe* summed it up as "a delight, a novel that travels seventy years of history on its sweet feet, a book of love and wisdom and irony."[2]

The declared subject of the novel is recollection of the cultural life of the city of Toronto, more specifically the small area around the Anglican church of St. Aidan. There are several narrators, of whom the principal one is Dr. Jonathan Hullah, an erudite physician whose approach to practicing medicine is influenced by the writings of Paracelsus, Robert Burton, Sir William Osler and Carl Jung. Osler considered Robert Burton's *Anatomy of Melancholy*, frequently referred to in the text, as the "greatest book of psychiatry that had ever been written by a layman."[3]

Dr. Jonathan Hullah, a diagnostician in private practice and a professor on the faculty of Medicine, has a reputation of successfully treating difficult chronic diseases, although his colleagues often distrust his therapeutic methods. His urge to become a physician was strongly influenced by an episode from childhood when, at the age of eight, he had scarlet fever and was so gravely ill that the local physician, Dr. Ogg, who was more bootlegger than healer, feared that he would not survive. He recovered and attributed the cure to an Indian woman, Elsie Smoke, an herbalist. She set up a tent in the yard of his house and performed rituals, after which he had a crisis followed by recovery. He tried in vain to discover who Elsie's "helpers" were in her supplications. As a youngster he often hung around Dr. Ogg's office, helping him mix tonics and prepare salves for his local patients, predominantly metis (people of mixed race) and Indians. The tonics contained rhubarb, senna and cheap red wine, and the salves for rheumatic ailments were a mixture of Vaseline and oil of wintergreen, which produced heat and a strong healing smell.

In medical school he fell under the spell of psychoanalysis, becoming a Freudian fanatic, which helped him develop a habit of careful observation that grew with the passing years. Subsequent service in the army during the war and experience as a police surgeon, in the coroner's office and in the emergency room have taught him to understand all classes of society and have provided ample exposure to human misery and vice. He believes that each physician is to some degree a psychiatrist and values the importance of talking with his patients, such as the wounded soldiers who gratefully listen to a friendly, non-patronizing or foolishly simple talk, liking best a trust-inspiring conversation. A challenging assignment at the end of the war to care for a group of seriously wounded victims of friendly fire prompted him to initiate a Reading Hour, posing a difficult choice of appropriate books for a largely uneducated audience. It was, however, a success. "The Raven" was the soldiers' favorite poem; they also liked Chaucer's "Miller's Tale" and Southey's "Bishop Hatto and the Rats".

One of the two lesbian ladies from whom he rented a flat and office space in a reconstructed stable on their property after the war described him as long and cornery looking, like a horse with a secret sorrow. He himself said that his face bore a certain morose splendor. At the very end of the war he became a victim of a nearly fatal accident, when he was trapped in a bathtub of filthy icy water for four days in a house hit by a V2 bomb in London. The uncertainty of whether rescue would come in time caused serious reflection on the identity of the prayed-to "helpers" who had saved him during childhood, a spirituality that meshed with his life. Exhausted physically and emotionally after his rescue, he did not expect to be up to par again and determined to live the rest of his life on his own terms. This meant that he wanted to be completely independent, to practice solo without haste, promotions, dependence on referrals or fear of losing practice to competition. Such an approach required not only wisdom but financial security, which he achieved by investing his inheritance well and becoming independently wealthy. His war experience made him mistrustful of medicine that prescribes a particular remedy for a particular set of symptoms. What he tried to avoid was the weariness and boredom of work that often led to *pro forma* treatment, especially with dull or unappealing patients.

Jonathan Hullah was broadly educated in many fields outside medicine, having discovered that real education meant things that you really wanted to know rather than things other people thought you should know. He observed that "doctors are men of substantial education, though not always men of wide culture."[4]

He remained single; the only big love in his life, from the time of their passionate affair in medical school, was an Irish gynecologist, Nuala, who married his best friend, Rocky Gillmartin, while Hullah was away during the war. Fortunately this was a woman who could love two men and had frequent occasions to travel from Salterton, where she lived, to Toronto to visit and console her former lover.

An unconventional physician, Hullah had a good memory and good hands, but was not a surgeon by nature, believing that surgery requires an extraversion of temperament that he lacked. If one had to apply a label to his expertise it would be as a psychosomaticist, but he never rejected conventional methods if he deemed them necessary. To quote him:

> Treatment must be intensely personal and if sometimes it strays into the realm of the mind, there the physician must follow it. But usually it is in the realm where mind and body mingle – where the mind affects the body and the body affects the mind, and where untangling the relationships is the Devil's own work, and takes time and application and sympathy – that the hard driven general practitioner and his specialist brothers cannot be expected to provide for every patient who knocks on the door.[5]

Hullah admitted that he could not do much for a patient whom he disliked. Psychotherapy, yes, but not psychoanalysis – admittedly a marvelous but extremely limited adventure in human understanding. He did not refrain from advocating another look at religion as a way to better health. He always claimed that he approached his patients intuitively, listening closely to every hint of body and speech. This was how he justified not forbidding the brandy and pipe his good friend and patient so thoroughly enjoyed, even though these addictions would probably be injurious to him over time.

He had a well-equipped, comfortable office with an elegantly furnished reception room and several examining rooms, where he was aided by his Danish secretary-nurse-masseuse-hydro-pathologist-and-general-healer, Frau Inge Christofferson. There was also a young physician assistant in training. Doctor Hullah willingly made house calls, from which he learned things about his patients that he would not have discovered during office visits. He wanted to know how his patients lived, to see their bedrooms, bathrooms and kitchens. "A whole world of habit, cast of thoughts, approach to health, approach to sex – all can be read in a bathroom."[6] He derived information from the smell of the house, insisting that he could smell disease, disquiet and unhappiness. He believed strongly that "the doctor who refuses to make house calls cannot hope for any sort of medical awareness."[7] His practice was best described by his landlady in a letter to her friend, the sculptress Barbara Hepburn in England. (The recipient is probably a real person, since a sculpture by an artist of that name is exhibited in the Indianapolis Museum of Art.) "The patients are of all kinds – invalids, young people looking worried, poor people, rich people with expensive cars, mostly women but a good sprinkling of men."[8]

Many doctors referred to him when their patients had exhausted their own endurance; then Hullah became a sort of a Court of Last Resort. One such patient was Miss Fottergill, a rich 53-year-old spinster whose main pre-occupation, after having spent the best years of her life nursing her selfish and intolerant mother, was to enjoy her own ill-health. Having exhausted and worn out the patience of several physicians who found her intolerable, they collectively shifted her to Dr. Hullah, who assessed her as a sexually frustrated woman lacking friends and having no sustaining interests in her life.

His landlady's letter contained an amusing description of how this patient, after being stripped naked by the nurse, was subjected to an hour-long examination by Dr. Hullah, who, after shaking hands, stared at her a long time, poked her in different places, turned her around and sniffed the area that she described as "You Know Where." After this, the treatment prescribed for her consisted of such measures as massage, steam bath, oatmeal bath and needle showers. The effects were spectacular. Miss Fothergill declared that Dr. Hullah was the first physician who bothered to understand the true nature of her ill health. Thus he became the object of her enthusiasm and platonic affection because he took the time to listen to her; indeed, she became his trumpeter. For his part, Dr. Hullah felt that he had done her a lot of good by "setting her squarely in the sort of health she desired,"[9] which happened to be a case of mild chronic rheumatoid arthritis.

Most intelligent physicians learn to realize that there are illnesses curable by scientific means, that some are incurable, that many discomforts will disappear without treatment and that the majority of non-life-threatening ills of the body either originate in the mind or are strongly affected by the patient's state of mind. The essence of psychosomatic medicine is to unravel this connection and help the patient obtain release. Hullah used many innocent tricks, such as giving a patient an elixir containing some innocent ingredients with a label saying that the prescribed dosage must never be exceeded, even though a gallon of the stuff could be imbibed with impunity. Thus he acquired a reputation of a pragmatist, a humanist, a man able to see through a brick wall. Others called him a cunning man, but he always maintained that the more he saw of illness, the less he knew.

In the final section of the novel, Dr. Hullah, now 65, decides to give his life fresh interest by engaging in a new form of literary criticism. He will "apply modern medical theory to the notable characters of literature and call the resulting book *The Anatomy of Fiction.*"[10] He will analyze the writing of novelists to diagnose the illnesses and causes of death of various literary heroes. For example, Falstaff died of alcoholic cirrhosis of the liver, with jaundice and ascites.

Although a dedicated physician throughout the story, Hullah's life is more varied and intellectually challenging than that provided by medicine alone. Among his friends and acquaintances are journalists, lawyers, musicians, artists and clergymen – a cast of characters playing various roles in the ingenious plot. There is even an unsolved mystery, when Father Menian Hobbes drops dead serving mass on the High Altar of St. Aidan Episcopal Church on Good Friday and Hullah remarks that the story would have been different if only he had taken the poor priest's false teeth for forensic examination.

We will not reveal the explanation of the mystery to potential readers, but it is not as wondrous as the portrayal of Dr. Hullah's medical practice, which is presented with remarkable insight and precision by a writer who is not a physician.

## REFERENCES

1  Davies R (1994). *Cunning Man.* New York: Penguin USA; 1994.
2  Penguin Group USA. The Cunning Man. *Book Clubs/Reading Guides.* Available at: http://us.penguingroup.com/static/rguides/us/cunning_man.html
3  Penguin Group USA, op. cit. From at interview with Robertson Davies.
4  Davies, op. cit., p. 216.
5  Ibid., p. 247.
6  Ibid., p. 258.
7  Ibid., p. 259.
8  Ibid., p. 273.
9  Ibid., p. 283.
10  Ibid., p. 377.

## PART FIVE

# Dispirited doctors

# CHAPTER 17

# *Ward No. 6 and Other Stories*

## by Anton Chekhov[1]

---

### Themes

- Obstacles to effective medical practice in provincial Russia
- Varied profiles of doctors in short stories
- Prevailing nihilism and lack of vital energy among Chekhovian doctors
  (Note: *see* Chapter 22 for Chekhov's biography.)

---

## WARD NO. 6

At a charitable provincial hospital there is an attached small pavilion reserved for mental patients, which is surrounded by weeds and has a rusted roof, a falling chimney and rotting wooden steps leading up to the front porch. The common room is filled with junk – mattresses, torn hospital gowns, underwear, worn-out shoes. There is unbelievable clutter and a suffocating stench. This is the command post of Nikita, the guard, an old soldier with a coarse face like a sheepdog and low brows. He is short and muscular, obtuse and simple-minded. He imposes order and maintains discipline by regularly beating patients with his strong fists.

There is one large ward. The walls are painted a dirty blue, the ceiling is smudged with smoke from the stove, there are iron grilles on all the windows and the gray floor is full of splinters. The place smells of stale cabbage, lamp oil, bedbugs, ammonia. The beds are attached to the floor and patients sit or lie on them. They wear loose blue hospital gowns and hats that resemble dunce caps.

Five mental patients live here. The first has TB, obsessively looks only in one direction and soon will die; the second is a lively little Jew who walks, sits, prays and laughs loudly. He went mad after losing his hat factory in a fire.

He is the only one allowed outside, where he begs for food and drink and a few kopeks, which are quickly taken away from him by Nikita. The third is Ivan Dmitrevich (Vanya) Gromov, a 33-year-old nobleman who suffers from a persecution mania and walks erratically about the room when agitated. He has high cheekbones and pale eyes that are mirrors into his tortured soul. He huddles in fear on a corner bed and his feverish talking reveals his insanity as he carries on about the miserable nature of mankind, the violence, the absence of justice and the stupidity and cruelty of his perceived tormentors.

Vanya's father was a respectable citizen before he was convicted of embezzlement and died in prison of typhoid. His possessions were auctioned off, leaving his wife and son penniless. Vanya had studied at the university and had a good job, but after the family disgrace he dropped out and worked as a tutor, schoolteacher and clerk at the court of justice. He had no friends and was contemptuous of most people because they lacked education and grace; he was a typical malcontent, but one who could see clearly the evils of society. He became obsessed with the idea that he would end up a convict and was sure he'd be accused of murder when two bodies were found in a spring near the cemetery. He finally became obviously insane with paranoid delusions and was committed to this hospital. Of the other two patients, one is a peasant who is regularly beaten by Nikita, the other a former merchant harboring a secret. Their routine is monotonous – morning tea, cabbage soup and kasha for midday dinner, leftovers at night. The only visitor is a barber who comes every two months.

Into this place of physical decay and human misery arrives Dr. Andrei Efimovich Ragin, a gentle man who wanted to be a priest but, obeying his father's wish, studied medicine, for which he has no calling. A heavy-set individual with coarse features who looks like a peasant, he has a stern face with a prominent network of little veins, small eyes and a red nose. He is tall, with broad shoulders and huge feet and hands, which could kill a man with one blow. Yet he moves slowly, cautiously, almost stealthily, always ready to yield to a passerby and to apologize in a soft flat voice. A small swelling on his neck prevents him from wearing stiff starched collars; instead he puts on soft linen or cotton shirts. He does not dress like a doctor. He wears the same suit for 10 years and, if he buys a new one from a Jewish haberdashery, somehow makes it look old and wrinkled almost at once. He dons the same jacket when he visits patients, eats dinner or goes to visit acquaintances. This is not because he is stingy; rather, he is completely indifferent to his appearance.

When Andrei Efimovich Ragin was appointed to head this charitable institution, he found it in a state of desolate disrepair. The stench emanating from the building and courtyard was suffocating; the spouses and children were sleeping with the patients and enduring bedbugs, cockroaches and rats. The operating room was inadequate, there were only two scalpels and not a single thermometer, and the bathtubs were used to store potatoes. The administrator, supervisor and felcher (physician's assistant) robbed the patients. The doctor who preceded Andrei Efimovich had been selling the hospital's alcohol allotment and was rumored to have had a harem of women recruited from patients' families and nurse's aides. The town population knew about this state of affairs, even exaggerated it, but was indifferent because the conditions of their homes were not any better. They joked that you do not go to the hospital to feast on pheasants and, besides, this is about all that the town can afford.

After investigating the hospital, Andrei Efimovich thinks that the best course would be to send the patients home and close down the facility, but he does not believe that he can accomplish this alone and knows that it would only transfer the corruption to another location. He rationalizes that if such misery and moral decay exist it means that they have a purpose and will eventually be transformed into something useful, the way dung finally becomes fertile soil. Thus the new chief changes little. He asks the families and nurses' aides not to stay overnight in the patients' room and installs two new cupboards with instruments, but he does not remove the administrator, the supervisor or the breeding sites of erysipelas (strep infections).

Andrei Efimovich is an honest man who believes in justice but lacks the strength to impose his will. He does not know how to give orders, how to insist on their execution, how to forbid bad practices. He never raises his voice or gives commands and is incapable of firing someone or making anyone stop stealing. When he receives a voucher with falsified accounts, he is embarrassed and guilty but signs it anyway. When patients complain of hunger or brutality, he is again embarrassed and mumbles something about a possible misunderstanding that he would try to clarify later.

At first Andrei Efimovich works diligently, sees patients from morning till night, operates, delivers babies and acquires the reputation of a good diagnostician, particularly for women's and children's illnesses. But with the passage of time the work becomes tedious and seems purposeless. The more patients he sees, the greater are the numbers of new and returning patients, while the town's mortality rate remains unchanged. He concludes that by seeing 12,000 outpatients a year his only accomplishment is to deceive 12,000 people. He cannot hospitalize the seriously ill and treat them properly because he lacks clean, well-ventilated facilities, nutritious food and adequate help. He is defeated by the terrible conditions – the filth, the stench, the rotten food. And why, he asks himself, should one interfere with the process of dying if death is a normal event in everyone's life? What is accomplished by helping a salesman or scribe live five or 10 years longer? Why should suffering be alleviated if, as it is said, suffering improves character? If the practice of medicine relieves suffering, he reasons, then those no longer suffering will only stray from religion and philosophy, which are the only true sources of happiness. Pushkin suffered horribly before dying and Heine was paralyzed for years before his death. So why should ordinary men and women escape it? Wouldn't their lives without a measure of suffering be as empty and meaningless as the life of an amoeba? Rationalizing like this, Andrei Efimovich stops making daily rounds at the hospital, staying home instead and reading.

He can visualize the hospital scene even when he is not there: a dark, narrow corridor for outpatients, with peasants in heavy boots, uniformed practical nurses, people in hospital gowns, crying children, orderlies carrying dead bodies and basins with excrement. He knows how hard this is on febrile, consumptive or sensitive patients but what can he do? When he does go to the hospital he encounters the felcher, a pudgy man with a clean-shaven face and soft movements, who is overwhelmed with work while the doctor does little – he has stopped operating because he cannot bear the sight of blood. Sometimes he dispenses ointment or castor oil. If he tries to examine a child's throat and the child cries, the doctor becomes dizzy and nervous and waves the youngster away. He is annoyed by all the confusion and, after seeing five or six patients, goes home to his office and starts reading. He spends half of his salary on books, mostly history and philosophy. He subscribes to one medical journal but only looks at the index. He reads slowly, stopping to contemplate passages that are difficult to comprehend. In front of him sits a decanter of vodka and a pickle; every half hour he pours himself a glass of vodka and takes a bite of the pickle. At 3 p.m. he asks the cook to serve his dinner. After a bad, sloppily prepared meal, he paces the room and meditates. Sometimes in the evening the postmaster comes for a visit. This man used to be a wealthy landowner and a cavalry officer but, after losing his estate, was forced to find a salaried job. The two friends smoke, drink beer and deplore the low intellectual level of the townspeople, who lack interest in the higher spiritual aspects of life. After his friend leaves, the doctor resumes his reading. He is fascinated by the highly differentiated brain centers of human intelligence and creativity and puzzled by the orderly process which puts an end to life, transforming a live body into dead matter. There is little comfort knowing he will be changed into some other organic form. He suffers from insomnia.

Meanwhile the town has made available funds to increase the hospital staff and hires another physician to help the doctor, Eugene Fedorovich Chobotov, a young man not yet 30, a tall dark-haired individual with widely set small eyes, probably of foreign descent. He arrives without a penny but with a small suitcase and a young, unattractive woman, who carries an infant and whom he presents as his cook. The new doctor establishes a close relationship with the felcher and the administrator. He possesses only one book, a set of the newest prescriptions from the Clinic of Vienna (1881), which he always takes along when visiting patients. In the evening at the club he plays pool but does not like cards. He speaks in intellectual-sounding clichés. He visits the hospital twice a week, makes rounds and sees outpatients. The complete absence of sterile technique and the blood-drawing cups raise his indignation, but he does not change the established order, not wishing to offend Andrei Efimovich, whom he envies and suspects of being a cheat and making a lot of money from this medical enterprise. Chobotov wants his job.

One day, almost by accident, Andrei Efimovich enters the psychiatric pavilion and encounters the agitated Ivan Dmitrievich, who asks him why he is being confined when hundreds of insane people walk free? Is the medical profession competent to tell a sane from an insane man? The doctor admits that it is a pure accident.

"Then let me go," insists Ivan.

"I cannot. If I do the police will catch you and return you to the institution."

"This is true," admits Ivan.[2]

The open, intelligent face of Ivan Dmitrievich evokes pity and compassion. The doctor sits down on his bed and starts a friendly conversation. He learns that Ivan attended university and is a well-read, intelligent and sensitive man who is aware of his paranoia. Dr. Ragin enjoys this patient's company and counsels him to ignore the grim surroundings and seek inner peace. They have philosophical discussions on a high level and Ivan tells the doctor that he knows nothing about suffering and says that his philosophizing and contemplations represent laziness and indolence. This does not upset Dr. Ragin. He is delighted and congratulates his patient on his correct assessment and begins to visit Ivan on a regular basis; the visits become longer, the conversations more passionate. They discuss philosophy, religion, human suffering. The doctor admits that his new friend is the most intelligent and interesting conversational partner in town. As their debates become more heated, the hospital personnel begin spreading gossip that the doctor is losing his marbles. A commission is appointed to examine his sanity and he is retired.

The postmaster takes him on a trip to Moscow, St. Petersburg and Warsaw. But Andrei Efimovich has no interest in sightseeing and spends the days lying on a couch in the different hotels where they stay. He gives his money to his friend, who loses it playing cards, so he returns to town without money or a job. He moves to a cheap, rundown flat where he vegetates. Without the means to subscribe to journals he loses interest in reading and sits peeling potatoes and sorting grain for gruel. He goes to church on Sunday and listens to the chants, reminiscing about his parents, his university days and religion. A few times he visits his friend in the psychiatric pavilion but he is too dejected and angry to pursue the conversation.

Lying on the couch he mulls over the injustice of being fired after 20 years of service without a pension or severance pay. He feels that he has not performed well but that does not justify denying him a pension. Destitute and dejected, he owes money to the landlord and grocer. His two visitors, the doctor who took his job and the postmaster who squandered his savings, treat him as though he is slipping into insanity and hospitalize him to sedate him with bromide. But one day, listening to their blabbering, the doctor loses his patience, insults his visitors and kicks them out, throwing his glass with the bromide against the wall. After they leave he is shaking feverishly, repeating incessantly: stupid people, stupid people. Later he cannot sleep and the next morning he goes to apologize to the postmaster. But his friends have already decided his fate. Under the pretext of a consultation, his successor brings Andrei Efimovich to the hospital and leaves him in the pavilion for the insane, where Nikita makes him undress, takes away his clothes and gives him some ill-fitting rags to wear. He is locked up in the asylum. When he realizes what has happened he demands to be freed but Nikita savagely beats him. The next day he has a stroke and dies. His funeral is attended only by his old cook and the postmaster.

## OTHER CHEKHOVIAN DOCTORS

In *Ward No. 6*, when Doctor Ragin ceases to attend to his duties and spends most of his time reading philosophy and religion, he no longer follows the medical literature. This attitude might have reflected Chekhov's personal dilemma of sacrificing his medical practice to writing fiction. He returns to this subject in a short story, *Grasshopper*, featuring Dr. Dymov, a decent, good-natured man and a dedicated physician with an inquisitive mind. His busy schedule is divided between patients and research in pathology, and he is highly respected by his peers. But he is ignored, ridiculed, exploited and deceived by his young bride, who, akin to a grasshopper, jumps around in a circle of artists, painters and musicians, a motley crew fond of wining and dining in Dymov's house without paying attention to the host. Dymov ends up dying at the age of 32 after aspirating a tracheal secretion from a patient with a malignant form of diphtheria. This could have been accidental or due to negligence, or perhaps it is a voluntary exodus from the humiliation and deceit of his disastrous domestic situation.

Shortly after the impulsive wedding of this incompatible couple, Dymov was reproached by his wife for having no interest in music or painting. He replies:

> "I don't understand them; I have spent all my life working at natural science and medicine and I have never had time to take an interest in the arts. Your friends don't know anything of science or medicine but you don't reproach them with it. Everyone has his own line."[3]

In another story, called *A Doctor's Visit*, Dr. Korolyov is sent by his superior to the countryside to see a factory owner's daughter who is ill with heart palpitations. He finds nothing wrong with Liza's heart and says:

> "The heart is all right . . . it's all going on satisfactorily; everything is in good order. Your nerves must have been playing pranks a little, but that's so common. The attack is over by now, one must suppose; lie down and go to sleep."[4]

He says that the factory doctor is perfectly competent to treat her. Yet he is so touched by her deep sadness that, when her distraught mother begs him to stay overnight, he unwillingly agrees, thinking about all the work that awaits him in Moscow. He spends most of the night wandering about, speculating on the factory buildings and the sad lives of the owners, managers and workers. Finally, he has a longer talk with his patient, who says she is weary and frightened and has no close friend to talk to, that she spends all her time reading when she is not worrying and ill. He thinks a husband is in order but, unable to produce such a cure, he realizes what she needs is to get away. He suggests this obliquely as Liza wonders abstractedly where she might go.

Though today a doctor might see Liza as a depressive in need of Prozac, this mild suggestion is the be all and end all of Kornilov's doctoring. Thus he quickly joins these other rather sad Chekhovian doctors, who lack the will or ability to act decisively. Yet the writing is fine; in only 11 pages, Chekhov portrays realistically the vast countryside and the factories and acquaints the reader with Liza, her old mother, the governess and the doctor, who are real people coping with the vagaries of daily life.

In yet another story, called *Ionitch*, Dimitri Ionitch Startsev, a newly appointed district doctor, falls in love with the beautiful young daughter of a local socialite, nicknamed Kitten. He proposes marriage to her, but she, confident of her musical talent because she plays the piano, sings and acts, turns him down and goes to the Moscow Conservatory to seek fame, success and freedom.

Four years later Startsev has acquired a large practice in town. He has grown broader and stouter and is no longer fond of walking, as he has become asthmatic. His only diversions are playing cards and keeping track of his accumulating account in the Mutual Credit Bank.

Kitten, now called Katherine, has returned from Moscow. She is no less beautiful but has lost the look of childish naiveté, having discovered that her musical and acting talents are insufficient for a professional career. She would like to revive Startsev's feelings but he has lost interest in marriage and is in fact pleased that he did not marry her.

Several additional years pass. Startsev has grown stouter as a result of his excellent appetite and lack of exercise. He breathes heavily. His practice has become immense, but greed does not allow him to give up his work as a district doctor, and he attempts to be at several places at once. The rolls of fat on his neck have changed his voice, which has become thin and sharp. He is ill-humored and irritable. His lonely life without friends is joyless, and he has no other interests beyond amassing more property, which now includes an estate, two houses in town and a soon-to-be-bought apartment house, a promising investment. The story ends without revealing who might inherit this estate. Here is another sad, lonely doctor who is much more interested in collecting property than having a family or taking a broader interest in life.

Reading these stories one wonders whether much has changed in the depths of Russia over the last hundred years. Has the status and remuneration of doctors improved? Not much information can be derived from the press. In contrast to lively contacts with numerous medical participants from many other parts of the world, one seldom sees Russian scientists and doctors at international meetings in the West, even though there are no longer government-imposed obstacles to travel from Russia. One should hope that today Chekhov's stories about doctors and the kind of medicine they practiced at the end of 19th century are of historic interest only.

## REFERENCES

1 Coulehan J, editor. *Chekhov's Doctors: a collection of Chekhov's medical tales*. Kent and London: Kent State University Press; 2003, including *Ward No. 6* (1892), *The Grasshopper* (1892), *A Doctor's Visit* (1898).

2 Ibid., *Ward No. 6*. p. 110.

3 Ibid., *Grasshopper*. p. 138.

4 Ibid., *A Doctor's Visit*. p. 176.

# CHAPTER 18

# Physicians in the world of Graham Greene

*A Burnt-Out Case*[1]

*The Human Factor*[2]

*The Honorary Consul*[3]

---

### Themes

- Voluntary suffering is needed to comprehend the human condition
- Murder without remorse in service of the government
- A doctor unable to feel love or empathy makes the wrong choice of profession

---

Graham Greene was an influential playwright, novelist, travel writer and critic. Early in life he converted to Catholicism, from which he often transgressed in his personal life, but Catholic religious themes are at the root of many of his novels. Unlike his contemporary French Catholic writer François Mauriac, Greene was not awarded the Nobel Prize, though he was frequently nominated for it. He is a widely read author with a writing style that is readily recognizable – lean, realistic and unsentimental. He portrayed the internal life of his damned but salvation-seeking characters, creating interesting plots with suspense-filled adventures. On the whole, the world of Graham Greene is sordid, cheerless, drab and seedy. The gloomy men and women who succumb to despair drift into some kind of spiritual abyss, groping for the crumbs of religious grace to rescue a few shreds of their shattered dignity.

Greene traveled widely, wrote numerous travel books and, like the fictional Dr. Maturin in Patrick O'Brian's seafaring novels, spied for the British government all his life; in fact, Kim Philby, the Soviet double agent, was his boss at M16. He collected odd characters he met abroad for his fiction and compared them to those in Chekhov's work. For example, in his book *The Lawless Roads*,[4] he recounts the scenes from an escapade to the most southern Mexican provinces, which took place in the spring of 1938, where the destruction of churches and the persecution of Catholic priests exceeded in zeal and brutality what happened in the rest of the country. He used this to gather material for one of his best novels, *The Power and the Glory*. He writes, "Like the characters in Chekhov they have no reserves – you learn the most intimate secrets. You get the impression of a world peopled by eccentrics, of odd professions, almost incredible stupidities, and, to balance them, amazing endurances."[5]

The doctors appearing in the following three novels are not their main heroes but are nevertheless interesting.

### A BURNT-OUT CASE

Dr. Colin is a minor character in the novel *A Burnt-Out Case*, published in 1960. The hero of the story is Querry, a womanizer, world-famous architect and builder of modern Catholic churches. He relinquishes his successful professional career and female companionship and, having decided to burn all bridges to the past, seeks seclusion in a place as remote from civilization as humanly possible. In his search for a refuge he comes to a leprosarium in Central Africa (The Belgian Congo) but cannot escape being recognized. Entanglement in a banal plot of tragic-comic misunderstandings costs him his life.

During his short stay in the leprosarium, which spans the plot of the novel, Querry strikes up a friendship with Dr. Colin, who had arrived with his wife some 15 years earlier, at first merely to care for the mutilated and to isolate new cases. More recently, however, he is able to arrest the progress of the disease with a new drug called DDS. The doctor's wife has died and is buried in a local cemetery, where he intends to join her some day. The superficial sketch of Dr. Colin gives no clues to his grim determination to remain in this place. He is lonely and agnostic among the missionaries of the order providing spiritual care to the leprosarium. His modest salary and the cost of drugs are borne by the state, not sufficiently generous to pay for an adequate supply of blankets, mosquito nets and other essential items. In the primitive hospital some of the patients must sleep on the floor, and Dr. Colin begs government to build a new hospital, arguing that drugs are cheaper than coffins. There are still new cases to be detected and treated and there are patients, particularly children, dying of other diseases.

Querry is welcome as the designer of the new hospital with a children's ward, lavatories and a dispensary. Dr. Colin's dedication stems from some kind of stubbornness rather than heroism or idealism. Why does he choose a vocation like this? asks Querry. The answer is by accident, the accident of his temperament. Subsequently he admits, however, that the search for suffering and the remembrance of suffering are the only means to remain in touch with the whole human condition. Dr. Colin's ministration to the lepers is not an act of compassion, but an extension of his malaise in the emptiness of his bleak existence.

## THE HUMAN FACTOR

In this espionage tale, perhaps the most exquisitely structured of all Greene's novels, we encounter Dr. Percival, a stout little rosy man in tweeds, overindulging in food and alcohol and conversing about fishing and modern painting. He is a former general practitioner, recruited by Her Majesty's Secret Service. The story revolves around a security leak in the African section of the Service. The leak is rather minor, mostly economic, but it happens in the aftermath of the shock wave following the sensational defections of Burgess, McLean, Philby and other Soviet spies, which had shattered the confidence of the British security system. Thus it was felt that the public should not hear about another security leak, particularly from such an insignificant outfit as this African section.

Exposing the mole does not appear to be a difficult task, because the section is manned by only two officers. The older of the two, Castle, had joined the Service more than 30 years before in South Africa. He is married, has a record of proven loyalty, is settled in his habits, is approaching retirement age and appears to be beyond suspicion. Such is not the case with his younger assistant, Davis, who is single, is somewhat eccentric, has a flair for gambling, a fondness for whisky, and is known to stuff absentmindedly into the pocket of his mackintosh some documents which, according to regulations, must be kept in a safe. There is not much hard evidence against Davis, but suspicion mounts when, under the pretext of a visit to his dentist, he sneaks into the zoo for a date with a secretary and manages to shake off the agent spying on him. His superiors in the Service agree that there should be no arrest, no trial and no publicity. The task of dealing with Davis is assigned to Dr. Emmanuel Percival, a senior man in the Service and a liaison officer with the bacteriological warfare department. Dr. Percival's medical knowledge is certainly out of date; he does not practice much, since taking care of the health problems of the department personnel requires little more than occasional checking of blood pressure. Besides, he is more interested in their working habits and loyalty than in their health. In the case of Davis, Dr. Percival is convinced that he should be eliminated quietly, peacefully and, if possible, painlessly, the way the Borgias got rid of their enemies. It seems natural to arrange a medical checkup, at which Dr. Percival finds that Davis has high blood pressure and a liver problem that he attributes to alcohol. The good doctor takes care of these problems and the unsuspecting Davis is grateful for the attention.

Dr. Percival is anxious to carry out an experiment using aflatoxin, a highly toxic substance liberated by a mold formed on rotten peanuts, because tiny doses of aflatoxin destroy liver cells in experimental animals. After ingestion mice rapidly become lethargic, lose appetite and die. A post-mortem examination shows liver necrosis and engorged kidneys.

Although 0.5 milligrams should suffice, Dr. Percival gives Davis a slightly higher dose. Later he confides to his friend and immediate superior that a side advantage of this situation will be finding out how aflatoxin works in a human being. Aflatoxin acts faster than predicted and Davis is dead within a few days. When asked whether he has some qualms of remorse, Dr. Percival replies that to die in only a week is a happy fate. The autopsy shows liver failure attributed to alcohol abuse. However, it turns out that Davis is indeed innocent, because the spy is Castle. When told that he murdered the wrong man, Dr. Percival shrugs it off. Not murdered, he replies, it was an error in prescription. The stuff had not been tried before on a human being. Besides, Davis should never have been recruited, he says. He was inefficient and careless and drank too much. He would have been a problem sooner or later anyway.

It would have been difficult to suspect such abominable callousness upon encountering this jolly man, who looked like an old family doctor, with his silver-rimmed spectacles and a small rounded pouch, concentrating over the menu in his favorite restaurant. Later, the friendly doctor does not hesitate to blackmail the wife of the real defector, Castle, by threatening to deport her child. His conscience is as untroubled as those of the SS doctors in Nazi concentration camps. In both cases loyalty to the regime overrides the Hippocratic oath of *primum non nocere*.

### THE HONORARY CONSUL

Dr. Eduardo Plarr, the central character and tragic hero of this novel, is the quintessential outsider. Born to a Paraguayan mother and English father, he is not comfortable in either culture but understands them both.

The action of the novel takes place during one week in the early 1970s in a provincial city in Argentina, near the Paraguayan border. Plarr practices medicine there because he was not successful or comfortable in Buenos Aires, where he grew up with his spoiled and helpless mother after his father, who has joined the Paraguayan revolutionaries, sent them to safety in Argentina.

There are only three Englishmen in this never-named town: Plarr, an English teacher of disagreeable temperament and Charley Fortnum, the honorary consul, who, at 61, is an alcoholic embarrassment to the British embassy in Buenos Aires.

Plarr is persuaded by a boyhood chum, Leon Rivas, an ex-priest turned Paraguayan revolutionary, to reveal the route of the American ambassador, who is coming to visit the town. Rivas and his group intend to kidnap him and trade him for 10 political prisoners in Paraguay, among them Plarr's father. By mistake they capture Fortnum, who is important to no one – not the British, the Americans, the Paraguayans; not even to his bride, the ex-whore Clara, who is also Plarr's mistress and carries his child. Fortnum's major wish to survive is centered on this young woman, whom he loves, and the child he believes to be his own.

Dr. Plarr's outsider status starts with his very profession. There is no clear reason for his being a doctor other than the need to move the story along. He has no love of healing, no inherent sense of service, no intellectual excitement. We see him only once in his consulting room and then for the purpose of introducing Rivas, and there are only occasional references to his nurse's starched uniform. However, he does respect professional medical ethics. When Fortnum, who is being held by Rivas and his men in a shack, is shot trying to escape and Plarr is called to attend to him, he cannot give in to his desire to tell Fortnum that he is Clara's lover and the unborn child's father, not out of generosity or honor but because it was his "wounded body which stopped him, stretched out helplessly on the coffin lid."[6] To disturb a patient's mind would be unprofessional. Instead Plarr is kept prisoner by Rivas and his men.

Plarr's background makes him neither entirely Spanish nor English. Colonel Perez, the Argentinean policeman charged with finding the terrorists and their victim, tells Plarr that he is nearly one of them. When Father Rivas asks him whether he is English or South American, Plarr realizes he cannot answer.

But like Camus' *Stranger*, Plarr is unable to feel or to love. At the beginning of his affair with Clara he reflects on the difference between a whore and a society woman in a real love affair. The latter picks up her lover's habits and becomes like him, sharing his interests; but a whore remains a stranger. "Her body has been scrawled over by so many men you can never decipher your own signature there," thinks Dr. Plarr.[7] Committed to avoiding the theatrical phrase "I love you" in his affairs with women of his own class, he attributes whatever emotion he feels to loneliness, pride, physical desire, or even a simple sense of curiosity. Thus when Clara admits that she loves him, he is horrified. Love is more than the proverbial snare and chain; it is a claim he won't meet, a responsibility he refuses. When he remembers the mother's love of his childhood, he likens it to the threat of an armed robber.

But Plarr is not completely devoid of feeling. He cares about his father, which is how he became involved with Rivas' plot in the first place; he is pleased that his father would approve of his work in the barrios of the poor; he is guilty because his father would disdain the selfish, upper-class women with whom he occasionally has had love affairs, but he would like Clara. Slowly his envy of Fortnum catches up with him, not because of Clara or the child – he has both – but because of Fortnum's ability to love them. In the end he tries to save them all by appealing to Perez, whose soldiers kill him along with all the kidnappers.

Why must Plarr die? Because he cannot love, and such a life is worthless? So Greene seems to be saying. Sin as much as you want, but, goddamn it, feel something, remorse, then confess, then sin some more. Fortnum, 61, an alcoholic and a loser, does survive, but he cannot bear to have Clara touch him because she sheds not a tear over Plarr's death. Until he realizes that she is covering up her infidelity, that she really did love Plarr, only then can his feeling for her return. He concludes that in an affair of this kind it was the right thing to lie and feels not only relieved but overjoyed that someone he loved would survive and remain close to him.

This is how Greene ends the novel. For purposes other than examining doctors in literature, one would see this as a novel about love and its absence and also the political terrorism which forms the background of the novel. Dr. Plarr is clearly not a believer. Throughout much of his coincidental imprisonment with Fortnum and the terrorists, he is merely an observer, a deeply pessimistic one at that, who expects no good to come of this affair. Here we have a hero so cut off from everyone that he winces at the memory of his mother's affection and clearly does not love Clara. Yet, in the end, he tries to save the situation, perhaps because of some remaining feeling of friendship for Rivas, a lingering regard for his father and a genuine desire to get him released from prison. A singular and puzzling hero, perhaps, but not in the world of Graham Greene, where the complexities of love, faith and betrayal are essential ingredients.

## REFERENCES

1 Greene G (1961). *A Burnt-Out Case*. New York: Penguin Twentieth Century Classics; 1992.

2 Greene G (1939). *The Human Factor*. New York: Simon and Schuster; 1978.

3 Greene G (1973). *The Honorary Consul*. New York: Simon and Schuster; 1973.

4 Greene G (1939). *The Lawless Roads*. New York: Penguin Classics; 2006. pp. 21–2.

5 Ibid.

6 Greene, op. cit., *The Honorary Consul*, p. 235.

7 Ibid., p. 111.

## PART SIX

# Abortion

# CHAPTER 19

# Drs. Wilbur Larch and Homer Wells (alias Dr. Fuzzy Stone)

## in *The Cider House Rules*

### by John Irving[1]

---

### Themes

- Illegal abortion
- Unwanted children
- The unceasing search for biological parents

---

John Irving, born John Wallace Blunt Jr. in 1942, is a best-selling American novelist and an Academy Award-winning screenwriter. As a student at Phillips Exeter Academy in Exeter, N.H., he was a wrestler and an assistant coach of the Academy's wrestling program, and wrestling is featured often in his books and stories. He attended the University of Iowa Writer's Workshop and wrote his first novel, *Setting Free the Bears*, at the age of 26.

The breakthrough in his career came with the publication of *The World According to Garp*, a big international best-seller and a cultural phenomenon, which was made into a film starring Robin Williams in the title role. In his 12 engrossing novels Irving developed a uniquely inventive style, reminiscent of Günter Grass, which imparted instantaneous recognition of the author by his readers. His voice is exclamatory and provocative, processing reality within a world filled with violence, destruction and bizarre coincidences. The characters are often cartoon-like, manipulated as puppets on a string. Their exaggerated characteristics are expressed by a single defining trait and a favorite repetitive sentence. Irving delights in the company of eccentrics, oddballs, prostitutes and freaks. Some of his characters are dysfunctional and malicious adolescents forced to deal with absent or unknown parents. Their sexual variations include adultery, pedophilia, trans-sexualism, rape, incest, homosexuality and liaisons between older women and younger men. He owes his appeal to highly imaginative plots, with stories told within stories, usually set in New England. There is much bantering, bravado and humor disguising a serious social or cultural message confronting the reader. In an article in the *New York Times*, on June 28, 2005, Irving admitted that his most recent novel, *Until I Find You*, contains two personal experiences he never previously revealed publicly, his sexual abuse by an older woman at age 11 and the recent entry into his life of his biological father's family, making the emphasis in his novels on orphans and the search for parents all the more telling.[2]

## THE NOVEL

*The Cider House Rules* is a capacious novel set in northern Maine. It was made into a movie in 1999 starring Michael Caine as Dr. Larch. The main theme is abortion, and the two central characters are Dr. Wilbur Larch and his assistant, the orphan Homer Wells.

Dr. Larch was born in Portland, Maine, and attended Bowdoin College and Harvard Medical School. His father was a disreputable drunkard whose graduation gift to his son was a prostitute who infected Wilbur with gonorrhea, an event that inhibited him from physical contacts with women for the rest of his life. During his internship and early years of practice in Boston, he became deeply impressed by the unsanitary conditions and disastrous consequences of clandestine abortions performed by quacks on women turned down by licensed doctors, even if they were victims of rape or incest. After service in France during World War I, he moved to St. Cloud's in 1920, an abandoned Maine mill town at the site of a former logging camp, where he founded an orphanage, with himself as director and staffed by two nurses who called him St. Larch. The facility became a Mecca for unwed mothers, for whom he performed God's work delivering babies, advising women about birth control, housing orphans and preparing them for adoption. There was also the Devil's work, abortions on demand, because, for the women who sought help at St. Cloud's, he accepted their right of choice – either an orphan or an abortion, even though the procedure was illegal at that time. He believed that abortions spared the misery of growing up as an unwanted child.

The orphanage was financially supported by the state and donations. The deliveries of unwanted babies and abortions were free. His own needs were modest, as he never learned to swim or to drive and never left St. Cloud's or its vicinity.

Dr. Larch was also the chronicler of St. Cloud's. His entries always began with "Here in St Cloud's"; for instance: "Here in St. Cloud's we treat orphans as if they were from royal families."[3] Accordingly, each evening when the children were in bed, he performed a benediction, addressing them as Princes of Maine and Kings of New England, followed by a 15-minute reading from Dickens's *Great Expectations* or *David Copperfield*. When a child was leaving to be adopted, he would add, "Let's be happy for one who found a family. Good night."[4] His own nights were spent in clouds of ether, to which he was addicted, but he learned to inhale an accurate dose so as to become alert when necessary and to disguise his habit.

Homer Wells (later Dr. Fuzzy Stone) is born in St. Cloud's orphanage in 1922. After all attempts to find him a family end in failure, he remains permanently at St. Cloud's as an apprentice to and a surrogate son of Dr. Larch. When a teenager, he is told by his mentor that he will finish medical school before starting high school. Indeed, not yet 20 years old, he absorbs *Gray's Anatomy*, the textbook of obstetrical procedures, and the content of Dr. Larch's notebooks from medical school. He dissects cadavers procured for him by Dr. Larch. On the practical side, he is a midwife to countless births and delivers many babies by himself. In an emergency, when Dr. Larch is absent, he successfully treats a difficult case of eclampsia.

Homer is also a surgical apprentice to many abortions but never performs one himself. He has an aversion to abortion, firmly believing that "You can call it a fetus, or an embryo, or the product of conception, but whatever you call it, it's alive. And whatever you do to it – you're killing it."[5] Believing that a fetus has a soul, he not only refuses to perform abortions but prefers never to watch them.

The beginning of another story within this novel takes place when Wallace (Wally) Worthington drives up in a Cadillac with his fiancée, Candy Kendall, to seek an abortion at St. Cloud's. Wally is the son of the Alzheimer's-afflicted owner of an orchard with a cider mill near the ocean, north of St. Cloud's. This is also the start of Homer's attraction to the couple, who invite him to leave St. Cloud's with them to work in the orchard and the cider house. There Homer will stay for the next 15 years, to the chagrin and disappointment of the abandoned Dr. Larch. After Pearl Harbor, Homer is exempt from service because Dr. Larch inserted a non-existent murmur of pulmonary valve stenosis into his medical record. Wally enlists in the Air Force and is shot down over Burma, acquiring mosquito-born encephalitis in the jungle, which paralyzes his lower extremities and makes him sterile. During Wally's long absence,

Homer and Candy become lovers. On one occasion, Homer breaks the fourth rule from Dr. Larch's printed pamphlet:

> *COMMON MISUSES OF THE PROPHYLACTIC. 4. Some men stay inside their partners for a long time after they have ejaculated; what a mistake this is! The penis shrinks! When the penis is no longer erect, and when the man finally pulls his penis out of his partner, the prophylactic can slide completely off; most men can't even feel this happening, but what a mess! Inside the woman you have just deposited a whole prophylactic, and all those sperm!*[6]

Homer and Candy take off for nearly a year, ostensibly to help the war effort at St. Cloud's, where Wilbur Larch teaches Homer pediatrics and Candy delivers Homer's son, Angel, pretending that he is an orphan whom Homer adopted. Homer circumcises Angel, hoping this will be the only pain he will cause his son. When the paralyzed Wally returns home he marries Candy, and the trio, aided by Wally's mother, manage the orchard and rear Angel Wells.

On one occasion Homer's anti-abortion stance breaks down. When the 15-year-old daughter of the foreman of the orchard, who already has one child as the result of incest, is repeatedly raped and injured by her father and becomes pregnant again, Homer reluctantly performs the abortion. After the procedure, the infuriated young mother procures a sharp knife, mortally wounds her father and goes off into the world.

Dr. Larch metamorphoses Homer into a physician who will be able to succeed him at St. Cloud's with a two-pronged approach. Homer has taken high school courses and has studiously read medical journals while Dr. Larch has been creating his credentials. A sickly child at the orphanage named Fuzzy Stone died of respiratory failure many years ago but remained alive in the diaries of Wilbur Larch, who recorded that Fuzzy was adopted by a caring family, received a high school and college education, subsequently graduated from medical school and was trained in obstetrics. The appropriate documents, including a medical diploma, are in Dr. Larch's possession. Before his retirement, which is finally demanded by the Board of Trustees when he is approaching age 100, Dr. Larch receives a fictitious letter from Dr. Stone, who is engaged in missionary work in Burma, announcing his wish to return to the United States and apply for a position at St. Cloud's. The Board interviews the returned missionary, Dr. Stone, a graying and bearded imposter, none other than Homer Wells. His worn-out black medical bag bears the insignia FS, and upon review of his credentials, the Board appoints him as the obstetrician in residence and the new director of the orphanage. On the matter of abortion, Dr. Stone surprises the Board with his adamant conviction that it should be legalized, but as long as abortions are illegal he will uphold the law.

After Dr. Larch dies in his sleep of an ether overdose, the nurse Angela, who is the first person to find the body, announces to the attending children: "Let us be happy for Dr. Larch. Doctor Larch has found a family," and the children respond, "Good night, Dr. Larch. Let us be happy for Dr. Larch."[7]

Because of his long absence from St. Cloud's, Dr. Stone is recognizable only to the old nurses, who are delighted to keep the secret. They always believed that you can take Homer out of St. Cloud's but you cannot take St. Cloud's out of Homer, who is returning to pursue the God's work begun by Dr. Wilbur Larch.


## COMMENT

For his exquisite knowledge of medical vocabulary and medical procedures, the author credits his access to his grandfather's textbooks: *The Expectant Mother's Handbook, A Textbook of Obstetrics* and *Safe Deliverance*. This grandfather, Dr. Frederick C. Irving, was Professor of Obstetrics at Harvard Medical School for many years. He also received advice from the noted author-physicians Dr. Richard Selzer and Dr. Sherwin B. Nuland.

Is this a credible story? The answer is that it is not meant to be. Is this an interesting, affecting and thought-provoking novel? The answer is definitely yes, perhaps even more so because it belongs in the category of novels fit to be taught in literature classes. In particular, we would recommend it to medical professionals interested in the never-ceasing abortion controversy.


## REFERENCES

1 Irving J (1985). *The Cider House Rules*. Toronto and New York: Bantam Books; 1986.
2 Wikipedia. *John Irving*. Available at: http://en.wikipedia.org/wiki/John_Irving
3 Irving, op. cit., p. 71.
4 Ibid., p. 109.
5 Ibid., p. 169.
6 Ibid., pp. 401–2.
7 Ibid., p. 569.

# CHAPTER 20

# Dr. Henry Wilbourne

## in *The Wild Palms*

### by William Faulkner[1]

---

### Themes

- Fatal attraction destroys a doctor's principles and career
- Death after botched abortion

---

William Faulkner (1897–1962) was born William Cuthbert Falkner in New Albany, Mississippi, and later added the "u" to his surname, either as the result of a typing error at the Winchester Repeating Arms Company, where he worked for a short time, or because, when applying to serve in the Royal Air Force during World War I, he thought this spelling looked more British.[2]

When he was four years old the family moved to the nearby town of Oxford, where he lived on and off for the rest of his life. Oxford is the model for the town of "Jefferson", and the county containing this town is the model for his fictional "Yoknapatawpha County." Faulkner's roots in North Mississippi ran deep; his great-grandfather, William Clark Falkner, served as a colonel in the Confederate Army, founded a railroad, wrote several novels, among them the best-selling *White Rose of Memphis*, and was the model for Colonel John Sartoris in his great-grandson's fiction.[3]

In 1925 Faulkner lived for extended periods in New Orleans, where he hobnobbed with the literary crowd, which included Sherwood Anderson, Hart Crane, Ernest Hemingway, Robert Penn Warren and Edmund Wilson, all of whom published their work in *The Double Dealer*, to which Faulkner also contributed several essays and sketches. While in New Orleans, he published his first novel, *Soldiers' Pay*, in 1926.[4] In 1930 Faulkner purchased the antebellum home Rowan Oak in Oxford, Mississippi, where he and his family lived for the rest of his life. Ten years after the writer's death it was sold to the University of Mississippi, which maintains it as it was in Faulkner's lifetime.

William Faulkner is considered one of the most important "Southern writers." In the majority of his works the action takes place in his native state of Mississippi, and he is regarded as one of the most influential and, by some critics, perhaps the greatest American writer of the 20th century. Faulkner's "modernistic" style of writing employs the stream-of-consciousness technique reminiscent of James Joyce, commonly dubbed "Southern Gothic." While his work was published regularly from the mid 1920s to the 1950s, Faulkner was relatively unknown before receiving the Nobel Prize in Literature in 1949 for "his powerful and unique contributions to the modern American novel."[5]

Some of the most celebrated of Faulkner's novels include: *The Sound and the Fury* (1929), *As I Lay Dying* (1930), *Light in August* (1932), *Absalom, Absalom* (1936) and *The Unvanquished* (1938); in all he wrote 19 novels. He also wrote over 100 short stories, often set, as are many of his novels, in the fictional Yoknapatawpha County. For his last novel, *The Reivers* (1962), he was awarded the Pulitzer Prize posthumously. This was his second Pulitzer, after receiving the first for *A Fable* in 1955. *The Reivers* also won a National Book Award that same year, his second; the first was for *Collected Stories* in 1951. In addition, Faulkner published six poetry collections and received credit for six of his screenplays, among them *Gunga Din*, *To Have and Have Not* and *The Big Sleep*. During his years in Hollywood he repeatedly collaborated with film director Howard Hawks.

Throughout his life Faulkner had a serious drinking problem, but he did not drink while writing. Among the pressures bearing on him were never-ending and maddening financial straits.

## *THE WILD PALMS (IF I FORGET THEE, JERUSALEM)*

This is a strangely structured book. Written in 1939, it contains two inexplicable and unconnected titles and relates two stories in which the characters, subjects and time of action bear no relation to each other. It is told in alternating chapters of a story called *Wild Palms* and one called *Old Man*.

In *The Wild Palms* story the time is 1937. The protagonist, Henry (Harry) Wilbourne, is a medical doctor and a graduate of a respectable medical school who is four months short of completing a two-year internship at a reputable hospital in New Orleans. At a New Year's party in the French Quarter, Harry meets Charlotte Rittenhouse, a woman with penetrating yellow eyes, who is married to a well-to-do, loving husband and is the mother of their two small children. There is an inadequately explained, instantaneous, irresistible physical attraction between Harry and Charlotte. Harry finds a wallet with $1200, burns the owner's identity papers, pockets the money and elopes with Charlotte, who abandons her family without a moment's hesitation. The adventure launches them on a self-destructive course while journeying through Chicago, Wisconsin, Utah and San Antonio and ending on the Mississippi Gulf Coast. They undergo a complete physical and psychological disintegration, which culminates in a botched abortion performed by Harry during the fourth month of Charlotte's pregnancy. Prior to this, Harry had done a successful illegal abortion on the wife of a foreman in a Utah mine. When Charlotte starts bleeding profusely, Harry awakens another nearby Mississippi doctor seeking his help, but he can do nothing and Charlotte bleeds to death. Witnessing the situation, this doctor telephones the sheriff, telling him to arrest Harry, who confesses to first-degree murder. A hostile jury sentences him to no less than a 50-year jail term. Before being taken to prison, Harry has the opportunity to end his life with a cyanide capsule handed to him by Charlotte's husband, but he turns it down.

Throughout the novel Faulkner uses a feverish stream-of-consciousness writing style, sounding like a shrill and discordant musical passage, to reveal Harry's confused state of mind as he obsessively raves about memory existing "outside the flesh" and then ceasing to be at all, ending this confusing tirade and the entire story by declaring that if he must choose "between grief and nothing I will take the grief."[6]

Does Harry deserve such a fate? Throughout his studies poverty crimps his life, excludes him from social or cultural interactions and makes him a loner who must work after hours to afford a pack of cigarettes once a week. At age 27 he is a naive virgin unable to comprehend or resist the advances of the impulsive Charlotte, who is caged in her dull domesticity and frustrated by her passionless marriage. Harry's impression of women is reflected in his uncomplimentary inner thoughts, which indicate that he does not believe that women can or do think or understand the essence of the males they choose. He then abruptly compares the extremes of the "cold penuriousness of the fabled Vermont farm wife" with the "fantastic extravagance of the Broadway revue mistress"[7] as he goes on and on about women's use of money and jewels as a some sort of wager or game, which gives them a degree of respectability in their chosen environment, even insisting that a "love-nest" must follow preordained rules and practices. Frankly these tirades fail to make much sense. It is interesting that Faulkner's biographer, who often quoted in his book passages from *Wild Palms* to exemplify Faulkner's original style, revealed that the author's literary agent, Phil Stone, was critical of the book because it was verbose and obscure.

Harry's inexperience and passivity hinder his integration into the unfamiliar outside world and he is unable either to finish his internship or obtain a paying job in the medical profession. He is not prepared to deal with Charlotte's unwanted pregnancy and fails to convince her to bear his child, which she adamantly rejects. His willpower dissolves into paralyzing inaction as the pregnancy advances. The novel does not explain whether he initiated the abortion or if Charlotte herself inflicted the fatal injury. Nor does Faulkner discuss the legality or morality of abortion, only the shame and the guilt. The final result is that neither Harry nor Charlotte come through as real, so that the reader cannot feel sympathy or sorrow for them, only confusion and disbelief and wonderment that a writer of Faulkner's stature and accomplishments could produce such a tale.

The other story, *Old Man*, is about two convicts evacuated from the Parchman State Farm Penitentiary during the catastrophic 1927 Mississippi flood. Implied here is that Harry may have a chance to meet them there 10 years hence. The scenes from the flood are wildly dramatic and the fates of the convicts are tragic. The heroic prisoner in this story, who saves a pregnant woman perched in a tree during the flood, surrenders himself to the authorities only to be slapped with an additional 10 years of incarceration for an attempted escape; like Harry, he accepts the verdict without protest, perhaps as an inevitable act of fate.

In these two narratives, inexplicably thrown together in a novel, Faulkner appears to impart the idea that a frightened and self-loathing man is paralyzed into inaction, becoming unable to resist the forces pushing him into an abyss. But the stories are not convincing, because the hapless submission of the victims to the unjust verdict defies the natural instincts of self-preservation. It could be, however, considered as a metaphor for the submission to the crushing force of political dictatorship.

In the end, Faulkner's stream-of-consciousness style and the hectic turmoil of gushing prose peppered with symbolism will appeal to the tastes of only selected aficionados of this eclectic genre.

## REFERENCES

1 Faulkner W (1939). *The Wild Palms (If I forget thee, Jerusalem)*. New York: Vintage Books; 1990.

2 Padgett JB. *William Faulkner*. The Mississippi Writers Page, July 30, 2007, University of Mississippi English Department, August 3, 2008. Available at: www.olemiss.edu/mwp/dir/faulkner william/print.html

3 Blotner J. (1974). *Faulkner: a biography*. Jackson, MI: Jackson University Press of Mississippi; 2005. p. 117.

4 Ibid., p. 177.

5 Ibid., p. 523.

6 Faulkner, op. cit., p. 273.

7 Ibid., pp. 69–70.

## PART SEVEN

# Satirized doctors

# CHAPTER 21

# Satire from the 17th to the 20th century

## *The Flying Doctor*

by Molière[1]

## *The Doctor in Spite of Himself*

by Molière[2]

## *Pygmalion and Three Other Plays*

by George Bernard Shaw[3]

## *The Good Soldier Švejk*

by Jaroslav Hašek[4]

---

### Themes

- Doctors as butts of ridicule amid the pervading ignorance and ineffectiveness of medicine through most of early history
- Today the science of medicine has changed, so that satirizing doctors as phonies and charlatans has become groundless
- Breach of professional ethics when subservient to a murderous regime

---

## MOLIÈRE (1622–73)

Here it is appropriate to begin with the French playwright and actor Jean-Baptiste Poquelin (1622–73), known by his stage name Molière, the creator of modern French comedy and one of the great masters of this art in Western literature. Molière, who was descended from a prosperous bourgeois family, studied to become an interior decorator like his father, and also studied law, but at the age of 21 abandoned his social class to pursue a stage career. After two years his theater troupe became bankrupt and he spent four weeks in prison for default on debt. He resumed his theatrical career in a new company, which toured the provinces for 15 years, often staging his own plays, which showed a genius for mockery. Few pieces survive from this period. Afterwards he moved to Paris and performed in several theaters, including one in the Louvre, where he performed before King Louis XIV. It is possible that the patronage of the king allowed him to get away with much irreverence in his satires of the French bourgeoisie, upper class and established institutions while carefully avoiding a critique of the monarchy and the Church. In his 14 years in Paris, Molière wrote 31 of the 85 plays performed at his theater, including such refined masterpieces as *Tartuffe* (*Imposter*) and *Le Misanthrope*.

Molière was a keen observer of human folly. He indicted pomposity and hypocrisy, and physicians were some of the favorite butts of his mockery. He ridiculed them in at least five of his plays, depicting them as ignoramuses who speak distorted Latin to impress the public with their pseudo-erudition, dispensing clysters (enemas), leeching and bleeding as remedies to restore the perceived imbalance among the four "humors" (blood, phlegm, yellow bile, black bile). This image is based on real-life doctors who practiced during the 17th century. When it comes to diagnosis, the doctors always disagree. They feel that it is more important to follow the rules laid by the Ancients such as Hippocrates than to save the patient. Yet they are always out to make money and are really just charlatans without useful knowledge of medicine.

In an early one-act comedy, *Le Médecin Volant* (*The Flying Doctor*, 1645), Lucille, the daughter of the respectable citizen Gorgibus, fakes illness to escape a marriage arranged by her father, because she is in love with her young suitor, Valère, and wishes to marry him. Valère, helped by her father's niece, Sabine, persuades his valet Sganarelle (a name frequently used by Molière in similar circumstances) to impersonate a doctor who will examine Lucille. Sganarelle, masquerading as a doctor, introduces himself as follows:

> "Hippocrates has said – and Galen has confirmed it with many persuasive arguments – that when a girl is not in good health she must be sick. You are right to put your trust in me for I am the greatest, the most brilliant, the most doctoral physician in the vegetable, mineral, and animal kingdoms"[5]

Afterwards he requests a urine sample from the patient, which he drinks and is dissatisfied that she cannot squeeze out an additional drop. He proclaims:

> "This is scandalous, Monsieur Gorgibus, your daughter will have to learn to
> do better than this. She is one of the worst urinators I have encountered. I
> can see that I will have to prescribe a potion that encourages her to flow more
> generously."[6]

But when paper and ink are procured, the doctor confesses than he had no
time to learn how to write. When the anxious father fears that his daughter
may die, Sganarelle reassures him that she is not allowed to die without the
right prescription. Finally, after seeing the patient, who is complaining of pain
in the head and the kidneys, he declares:

> "We must attribute this to the interconnections between the humors and the
> vapors. For example, since melancholy is the natural enemy of joy, and since
> the bile that spreads through the body makes us turn yellow, and since there is
> nothing more inimical to the health than sickness, we may conclude with that
> great man that your daughter is indisposed."[7]

Sganarelle declares that the patient needs fresh air and must go to the little
house at the end of the garden, where Valère is lurking so that they can run
off together and get married.

In the play *Medécin Malgré Lui* (*The Doctor in Spite of Himself*, 1666)
Sganarelle, a poorly educated woodcutter and drunkard, is forced to play the
role of a doctor, which he performs with gusto. He convinces the father of a
young daughter, who pretends to have lost her speech, that his knowledge
will cure her of the noxious "humors" and vapors given off by the exhalations
arising from the seat of disease. This earns him a handsome honorarium and
he muses:

> "I may just stay in the profession for the rest of my life. It is the most satisfying
> trade you can find. Whether you cure or kill you always collect that fee. Nobody
> jumps at you for doing a shoddy job."[8]

Malpractice?

> "You can rip and hack the material any way you want. A shoemaker knows that
> if he ruins a scrap of leather, he will foot the bill himself, but in this trade it
> won't set you back a penny if you ruin a human hide. When you slip up you
> are not to blame. It is the fault of the corpse. And, best of all, the dead are the

most honorable, discreet people in the world. They never complain about the doctors who did them in."⁹

In the last of his plays, *Le Malade Imaginaire* (*Hypochondriac*, 1673),¹⁰ the protagonist Argan, a miser addicted to illness, is milked by the doctors and apothecaries for all he's worth. Being irked by these expenses, he conceives a plan to marry his daughter to a physician and thus have free medical care from his son-in-law. The chosen young dim-witted doctor clings stubbornly to ancient beliefs and refuses to acknowledge modern ideas, such as the circulation of the blood. He prefers to treat the common people because there is no need to worry about the results, whereas the rich are more difficult since they actually expect to be cured. Argan is persuaded by his brother that his addiction to doctors is bad for him because they are ignorant of the workings of the human body and therefore can do nothing to cure it. They will kill their patients with their best intentions.

For Molière himself the doctors of that epoch could do nothing as he lay dying from a lung hemorrhage caused by pulmonary tuberculosis, which occurred only a few hours after completing his acting performance in the above play.

## GEORGE BERNARD SHAW (1856–1950)

The world-famous playwright, critic of music, art and literature and social reformer George Bernard Shaw was born into a poor but genteel Dublin household. His father was an alcoholic and his mother a professional singer. At the age of 20 he moved to London and stayed permanently in England. His writing career began with a string of unsuccessful novels, but he flourished as a critic and political activist, becoming a leading member of the Fabian Society, a group dedicated to progressive politics. In the 1890s he was deeply influenced by the dramas of Henrik Ibsen and began writing plays for the stage, some of which were satirical comedies and some of which were not, such as *Arms and the Man* and *Candide*. By the turn of the century Shaw matured as a dramatist with such plays as *Man and Superman* and *Major Barbara*. In 1925, he was awarded the Nobel Prize for Literature for the play *Saint Joan*. In all, he wrote 63 plays. Although remembered mostly for his comedies, Shaw made the British stage a forum for considering moral, political and economic issues.

In 1931 he visited the Soviet Union and met Josef Stalin. In 1933 he came to America for the first time, and in 1938 he received an Academy Award (Oscar) for the screen play *Pygmalion*, which was later made into the musical *My Fair Lady* and performed after his death. Shaw was a pacifist and vegetarian who neither smoked nor drank alcohol. He died at the age of 94 from complications related to a fall from a ladder. An ardent socialist and reformer, he first became disillusioned with society during World War I, and at the very end of his life he expressed doubt about the sound judgment of the poorly comprehending masses, thus suggesting that for such a society "benign dictatorship" may be a suitable form of governing. In the Preface to *Heartbreak House*, he wrote:

> It is said that every people has the Government it deserves. It is more to the point that every Government has the electorate it deserves, for the orators of the front bench can edify or debauch an ignorant electorate at will. Thus our democracy moves in a vicious circle of reciprocal worthiness and unworthiness.[11]

### The Doctor's Dilemma (1906)

The action of this satirical play takes play in London, probably in 1906. The morning paper contains an announcement that Dr. Ridgeon has been knighted for his discovery of a cure for tuberculosis by inoculation with a substance that raises the level of opsonin in the blood. This substance allows the phagocytes to destroy bacteria. When the infected patient is in a positive phase, inoculation cures the disease, but the inoculation kills the patient when he is in a negative phase. Dr. Ridgeon can tell by examining a drop of blood which phase the patient is in and proclaims that this is the most important discovery since Harvey explained the circulation of the blood. The amount of the available inoculate is limited, and only one dose is still available at the onset of the play. Here is the doctor's dilemma – which life should be saved among two candidates. One is Louis Dubedat, a gifted young painter who creates authentic art but is deceitful, immoral, unscrupulous and monumentally selfish. The other is Dr. Blenkinsop, a decent, congenial, honest but dull and inefficient doctor who is useless to society. Dr. Ridgeon chooses to save Dr. Blenkinsop, which condemns the talented painter, not because he weighs the moral options but because he has fallen in love with the painter's young wife and hopes to marry her when she becomes a widow. Unfortunately for him, Mrs. Dubedat chooses to marry someone else.

This medically nonsensical plot gives the author an opportunity to display a gallery of doctors paying visits to Dr. Ridgeon to congratulate him on his knighthood. Dr. Schutzmacher explains how he assures his patients of "Cure Guaranteed":

> "You see, most people get well all right if they are careful and you give them a

little sensible advice. And the medicine that really did them good is Parrish's Chemical Food phosphates, you know. One tablespoonful to a twelve-ounce bottle of water, nothing better, no matter what the case is."[12]

Then comes a surgeon, Mr. Cutler Walpole, a smartly dressed, energetic, unhesitating man of 40. He believes that nearly all patients suffer from blood poisoning that can be cured by the excision of the poison-harboring nuciform sac. "The operation ought to be compulsory; it's ten times more important than vaccination."[13]

The next guest is the physician to royalty, Sir Ralph Bloomfield Bonington, who recounts how he contributed to Ridgeon's knighthood by using Ridgeon's method to treat the young prince for typhoid. On a different occasion he inoculated a typhoid patient with tetanus anti-serum and the tetanus patient with typhoid anti-toxin by mistake, and they both recovered – proof that in both cases the inoculation stimulated the phagocytes.

The savage satire of doctors in this play is not much different from Molière's 250 years earlier, as Shaw's doctors have the same obsession with treatments that cure all diseases, pretending to possess non-existent knowledge, being jealous of professional rivals and using jargon that is incomprehensible to laypeople. He reinforces his views in his preface to the play, which is longer than the play-script itself. Here, Shaw declares that:

> the medical profession . . . has an infamous character. I do not know a single thoughtful and well-informed person who does not feel that the tragedy of illness at present is that it delivers you helplessly into the hands of a profession which you deeply mistrust, because it not only advocates and practices the most revolting cruelties in the pursuit of knowledge and justifies them on grounds which would equally justify practicing the same cruelties on yourself or your children, or burning down London to test a patent fire extinguisher, but, when it has shocked the public, tries to reassure it with lies of breath-bereaving brazenness.[14]

Malpractice can never be proven because

> the only evidence that can decide a case of malpractice is expert evidence, that is, the evidence of other doctors; and every doctor will allow a colleague to decimate a whole countryside sooner than violate the bond of professional etiquette by giving him away.[15]

Shaw is most vociferous in his attack on vivisection, declaring that the medical code regarding it is simply criminal anarchism at its very worst.

Some of his final admonitions to the public are:

> Nothing is more dangerous than a poor doctor. Treat persons who profess to be able to cure disease as you treat fortune tellers. Make it compulsory for a doctor using a brass plate to have inscribed on it, in addition to the letters indicating his qualifications, the words: Remember that I too am mortal.[16]

But such rhetoric in the preface rings hollow and the sarcasm in the play is widely off target because Shaw is too intelligent and too well informed not to recognize the beneficial services performed by the medical profession. In a roundabout retreat he acknowledges that infections and the way to avoid them are better understood than they used to be; that in most cases the motives in choosing the career of a healer are unselfish; and that the medical profession, like other professions, consists of a small percentage of highly gifted persons at one end and a small percentage of all-together disastrous ignoramuses at the other. Between these extremes comes the main body of doctors who can be trusted to work in a disciplined manner.

As a socialist he deplores that some doctors are hideously poor while others, such as surgeons and the owners of private hospitals, are excessively rich. Unlike some of his later more serious plays, *The Doctor's Dilemma* is not likely to be returned to the contemporary theater repertory, but it can serve as a reminder that this was the last satire of medical knowledge which, in the rest of the 20th century, expanded beyond the boldest imagination to give society access to better health and a vastly extended life span. At the same time it does not mean that improved knowledge automatically improves the character of physicians. And to underline this point, we encounter an even more savage satire next.

## JAROSLAV HAŠEK (1883–1923)

This Czech writer produced only one unfinished book, *The Good Soldier Švejk*. Hašek was not a typical writer and not a typical Czech. The son of an impoverished schoolteacher who drank himself to death, with the equivalent of a high-school education from the Czechoslovakian Academy of Commerce, he gained a reputation of a prankster and hooligan with a penchant for vagrancy. Throughout his disorderly Bohemian life, he wrote short stories and newspaper articles for radical publications and was in trouble with the police because of his editorship of the anarchist journal *Komuna*. In 1915, he was drafted into the Austro-Hungarian Army and sent to fight the Russians, for whom the Czechs had more affection than they did for their Austrian rulers. He was taken prisoner in Galicia and joined a voluntary military unit drawn from the Czechs and Slovaks, which evolved into a Legion fighting the Germans. After the outbreak of the Russian Revolution, he became a member of the Bolshevik Party, but in 1920 he returned to Prague, now in the independent Czechoslovakia, and drifted back into his drunken vagabond existence of the pre-war years.

In 1921 he began assembling his notes from various episodes of his disorderly life, gathered in taverns, jail, a short stint in an insane asylum, the draft board, military service, war and captivity, and gave them all to his anti-hero, the good soldier Švejk. Before the outbreak of World War I, Švejk was discharged from the Austro-Hungarian Army with a certificate proclaiming him a patent idiot. He lived happily in Prague, making a living by selling pure-bred dogs, which he created by cutting the tails and trimming the ears of captured street mongrels. The character and the attitude of Švejk were so uniquely original that the word Svejkism was incorporated into the vocabularies of several central European languages in the same manner that we use the names of Don Quixote, Falstaff or Oblomov. It is not easy to characterize Švejk in a brief description. The closest figure from the recent past is the tramp portrayed by Charlie Chaplin – a little man caught up in the cogs of a bureaucratic machine and designing his own camouflage for protection. Playing the role of an imbecile, Švejk baffles his interlocutors with an angelic smile, puzzling comments or an anecdote totally inappropriate for the occasion, and each of his encounters ends with the exposure of the immense nonsense and stupidity of the civilian and military structure of the Austro-Hungarian monarchy and a powerful indictment of the ugliness of the war.

Hašek's writing is not well edited; it is often chaotic and uneven, and his sarcasm is exaggerated, so that comedy turns into slapstick, but this hardly detracts from the originality of this comic masterpiece. Unfortunately, the scholarly English translation by Cecil Parrott cannot give the reader the full flavor of this work. This is acknowledged by the translator himself, who explains that Švejk's language is Švejk himself and this defies an accurate translation. Hašek died when two-thirds of the planned book was roughly completed. An attempt by another author to finish it after his death was not particularly successful. Today the image of the good soldier Švejk has probably faded into oblivion outside of his native land, but after World War I this was one of the most popular and widely read books.

### The Good Soldier Švejk

Švejk met doctors when the world war broke out and his status of a certified idiot no longer protected him from avoiding the draft to rejoin the needed cannon fodder. His encounters with the draft board were disastrous. A panel of three psychiatrists probed his sanity by asking: Is radium heavier than lead? The answer: "Please, sir, I have not weighed it." Do you believe in the end of the world? The answer: "I would have to see that end first." And to the question how much is 12,897 times 13,863, he answered 729 without batting an eyelid. After that the medical experts certified that Josef Švejk should be sent to a psychiatric clinic to establish how far his mental state endangers the surrounding people. Of the lunatic asylum, his opinion was favorable because "everyone there could say what he pleased."

The next encounter with the medical profession was in the military hospital to which Švejk was brought when he complained to the draft board of inability to walk because of rheumatism in his knees. Several degrees of torture were prescribed by Dr. Gruenstein for the patients, nearly all true or suspected malingerers. The routine treatment was: 1) Strict diet, a cup of tea each morning and evening for three days; 2) Generous portions of quinine in powder; 3) The stomach is pumped out twice a day with warm water; 4) Enemas with soapy water and glycerin; 5) Wrapping up in a sheet soaked in cold water. These methods often achieved recovery from alleged ailments with readiness to return to duty, but for the recalcitrant rest, several military doctors arrived from the commission and, of 70 patients, declared all but two to be fit for duty. Among them were three patients dying of consumption. Švejk was sent to the garrison jail for perceived insolence.

With the last batch of doctors the satire ceases to be comic, because we no longer deal with ignorant doctors who heal, but with doctors recruited to execute the directives of the non-medical authority. In some countries we may find such doctors who are asked to assist with the execution of prisoners or doctors who are requested to examine prisoners before they undergo "severe" interrogation.

An extreme deviation from medical ethics and humanitarian tenets was exhibited by the Nazi doctors during World War II, who selected victims to be sent to the gas chambers or tested how long a subject can survive submerged in ice-cold water. Several books have dealt with this subject, among them William Styron's *Sophie's Choice*.

## REFERENCES

1 *The Flying Doctor* in *The Actor's Molière, volume 4. One-act comedies of Molière*. Translated by A Bermel. 3rd edition. New York: Applause Theater Books; 1992.
2 *The Doctor in Spite of Himself* in *The Actor's Molière, volume 2. One-act comedies of Molière*. Translated by A Bermel. New York: Applause Theater Books; 1987.
3 Shaw GB (1906). *The Doctor's Dilemma* in GB Shaw. *Pygmalion and Three Other Plays*. New York: Barnes and Noble Classics; 2004.

4 Hašek J. *The Good Soldier Švejk*. Translated by C Parrott. London: Penguin Books; 1974.

5 *The Actor's Molière, volume 4*, op. cit., p. 33.

6 Ibid., p. 35.

7 Ibid.

8 *The Actor's Molière, volume 2*, op. cit., p. 30.

9 Ibid.

10 Molière JB. *The Hypochondriac*. In *Moliere's Comedies volume 2*. Translated by H Baker and J Miller. London: Dent; 1961. pp. 469–71.

11 Shaw, op. cit., Preface, p. 481.

12 Ibid., p. 255.

13 Shaw, op. cit., p. 265.

14 Ibid., Preface, p. 227.

15 Ibid., Preface, p. 170.

16 Ibid., Preface, p. 244.

## PART EIGHT

# Doctors in dramas

# CHAPTER 22

# Doctors in the plays *Ivanov, The Seagull, Uncle Vanya* and *The Three Sisters*

## by Anton Chekhov[1]

---

### Themes

- Harassing doctor
- Bored and cynical physicians
- Frustrations of medical practice in provincial Russia
- Early environmental awareness

---

Anton Pavlovich Chekhov was born in Taganrog, Russia, in 1860 and died of pulmonary TB in 1904. During his short life he created a prodigious number of memorable works. His great plays, such as *The Seagull, Uncle Vanya, The Three Sisters* and *The Cherry Orchard* started a new movement of subtle psychological drama that influenced George Bernard Shaw and other playwrights.[2] But before he became a famous playwright he wrote hundreds of sketches for newspapers; in fact, so apt were his descriptions of Russian street life and society it was said that if the country disappeared completely, it could be reconstructed from Chekhov's stories. In 1890 he traveled to the island of Sakhalin, north of Japan, to observe the conditions of Russian convicts there, publishing his findings in 1893, which greatly influenced subsequent penal reforms.

His family situation compelled his writing. In 1876 his tyrannical father, owner of a small grocery, went bankrupt and, with his wife and younger children, fled to Moscow to avoid debtors' prison. Chekhov stayed behind to finish his education at the Taganrog Gymnasium, supporting himself and his family with his writing, tutoring and catching and selling of goldfinches.

In 1879 he entered medical school in Moscow, graduating in 1884, thereafter dividing his time between the practice of medicine and writing, saying, "Medicine is my lawful wife, and literature is my mistress."[3] That same year he began coughing up blood but refused treatment, which would have been largely ineffective before the discovery of antibiotics. He took care of the poor without charge and never made much money from his medical practice. But his writing gradually evolved from sketches to short stories, which he started publishing in more prestigious literary journals. In 1887 he won the coveted Pushkin Prize for his short-story collection *At Dusk*.

Chekhov, known as Russia's most elusive literary bachelor, married late in life (1901) the actress Olga Knipper but only on the condition that they live apart, he at Yalta, she in Moscow. "Give me a wife who, like the moon, won't appear in my sky every day."[4] The advantage to history of this arrangement is a collection of their correspondence which contains gems of Russian theater history.

In addition to being one of the world's most admired playwrights, Chekhov is considered by many to be the greatest short-story writer who ever lived. (*See* Chapter 17 for a discussion of doctors in several of his short stories.)

## THE PLAYS

In most of Chekhov's plays there is a doctor in the cast but not in a leading role. For example, in the play *Ivanov*, the young doctor Lvov attends Anna, the wife of the protagonist, Nikolai Ivanov, and oversteps his physician's role by nudging Nikolai to take Anna, who is dying of consumption, to a warmer place in the Crimea and by incessantly chastising him for his callousness and indifference. A year after Anna's death, Ivanov is about to marry a wealthy young woman who is in love with him. Doctor Lvov steps in again, persecuting Ivanov with his accusation that he is marrying the woman for her dowry. The wedding does not take place, because Ivanov shoots himself, but it is not clear how much his conscience was rattled by the young fanatical doctor who was never paid for his visits to the unhappy Anna Ivanova.

In *The Seagull*, Dr. Dorn, a 55-year-old, well preserved, womanizing bachelor, takes care of the State Councilor Sorin, dispensing aspirin for everything that ails the old man. He is not a very comforting doctor, telling his patient, "But frankly taking medicine at your age, complaining you wasted your youth . . . well excuse me, but I think *that's* being silly."[5]

About himself he says: "I worked for thirty years without a break! I was always on call night and day, never had a minute to myself, all I managed to save was two thousand, and I spent that on a trip to Italy."[6]

At the end of the play, when the assembled company hears a shot outside, Dr. Dorn reassures everybody that it was a cork that popped out from a bottle in his medicine bag, but he knows that the failed young writer Konstantin has just shot himself.

In *Uncle Vanya*, Dr. Astrov, a handsome man in his mid-thirties, arrives ostensibly to treat the retired professor for gout, but he is more interested in the young wife of his patient. He is a very intelligent man but after 11 years of rural practice is bored and bitter. "I'm all worked out. I've gotten vulgar, my feelings are gone, I don't think I could have a relationship with another human being."[7]

He explains that at

> "Easter I had to go out to Malitskoye; there was an outbreak of typhoid fever. Those back wood shacks . . . the way those people are crammed in on top of one another; it was filthy! The stink, the smoke – they had livestock right in the same room with the sick people, pigs even. I ran around trying to help people, never stopped, did not eat a thing, got home that night – and you think I got any rest? They brought a signal man from the railroad yard . . . expected me to operate right then and there."[8]

It is truly remarkable that in a play written in 1896 Chekhov was acutely aware of man's impact on the environment. Dr. Astrov moans:

> "But our great woodlands are being leveled, millions of trees already gone, bird and animal habitats destroyed, rivers dammed up and polluted and all for what? Because we are too lazy to look for other sources of energy . . . the climate changing for the worse every day, the planet gets poorer and uglier."[9]

In a later monolog:

> "I could understand if in place of the trees we destroyed we had something. If there were communities, jobs, schools, then people might be better off, right, but none of that happened. We still have the same swamps, the same mosquitoes, the same poverty, the same diseases – typhoid, diphtheria. . . . What we are seeing here is the result of an uncontrolled struggle for survival. A man is freezing, hungry, sick, trying to save what's left of his life, trying to take care of his children, so what does he do? He lets instinct take over, he grabs whatever he thinks will feed him and keep him warm, he destroys everything around him without a thought for the future. It is almost all gone already, and there is nothing to replace it."[10]

For himself Dr. Astrov collects rare plant species and plants trees on his property. He does not succeed in luring Yelena, the professor's wife, to his home and does not respond to the advances of the professor's daughter, Sonya, who is secretively in love with him. When the professor and Yelena leave the estate and go back to the city, Dr. Astrov returns home, but from the amount of vodka he consumes in a single day one can see that he is already an incurable alcoholic.

In *The Three Sisters*, Dr. Chebutykin, an army doctor and one of three officers doting on the sisters, is a lonely, broken man one year away from his pension. He boasts, "I never have done anything, ever. Once I graduated I never did a single lick of work. I never read a single book."[11] Perhaps he could have gotten away with it as a doctor in the Russian Army. Dr. Chebutykin is a second in the duel in which the first lieutenant, Baron Tuzenbach, is killed a day before he was to marry one of the sisters. The doctor makes a heartless comment, asking what difference it makes.

In light of the portraits Chekhov paints of these medical men, one is relieved that there is no doctor in the cast of his last and most often performed play, *The Cherry Orchard*.

## REFERENCES

1 *The Plays of Anton Chekhov: a new translation by Paul Schmid*. New York: Harper Perennial; 1997.
2 Wikipedia. *Anton Chekov*. Available at: http://en.wikipedia.org/wiki/Anton_Chekhov
3 Ibid. Letter to Aleksei Suvorin, September 1888.
4 Ibid. Letter of March 1895.
5 *The Plays of Anton Chekhov*, op. cit. *The Seagull*. p. 128.
6 Ibid., p. 148.
7 *The Plays of Anton Chekhov*, op. cit. *Uncle Vanya*. p. 228.
8 Ibid., p. 210.
9 Ibid., p. 217.
10 Ibid., p. 236.
11 *The Plays of Anton Chekhov*, op. cit. *The Three Sisters*. p. 262.

# CHAPTER 23

# Dr. Thomas Stockman

## in *An Enemy of the People*

### by Henrik Ibsen[1]

---

### Themes

- Environmental clean-up clashes with economic profit
- Honest doctor defeated by his anger, stubbornness and self-righteousness
- Beware of the will of the majority

---

Henrik Ibsen (1828–1906) completed *An Enemy of the People* in Italy in 1882 when he was 54 years old, after he wrote *Pillars of Society*, *Ghosts* and *A Doll House* but before *The Wild Duck*, *The Lady from the Sea* and *Hedda Gabler*. In all, Ibsen wrote 12 great modern plays and is regarded as the father of realistic drama, which broke from the Victorian-era morality plays in which goodness brought happiness and evil brought pain. Ibsen looked behind the facades of society at the realities of human nature and behavior; thus his plays were revelatory and upsetting to his contemporaries because they shattered their firmly held illusions. This is not surprising given Ibsen's background and experiences. Though a descendant of several distinguished Norwegian families, his once-prosperous merchant father fell upon hard times shortly after his birth and became seriously depressed; his mother turned to religion for comfort.

Ibsen left home at 15 and became an apprentice to a pharmacist in the small town of Grimstad, seduced a local servant girl and, when she became pregnant, abandoned her. He went to Bergen, where he worked for the Norwegian Theater as a writer, director and producer. In 1858 he became the creative director of the Christiania (now Oslo) National Theater, married

Susannah Thoresen, fathered their only child, Sigurd, and struggled financially. In 1864 he settled in Italy, where he first achieved critical acclaim for his plays *Brand* and *Peer Gynt*. He was on his way to becoming the most influential writer in the European Theater.

## THE PLOT OF *AN ENEMY OF THE PEOPLE*

Thomas Stockman is a medical officer in the seaside resort town of Baths in southern Norway. In contrast to his brother, Peter, the mayor of the town, a rigid, pedantic, humorless and pompous man plagued by gastric ulcers, Thomas is jolly, outgoing, friendly and hospitable. He is loved and admired by his wife, his two sons and his daughter. Their house is open to friends and freeloaders, with whom he shares a hot toddy while puffing on his pipe. His own childhood was poor; he knew starvation and, later, the desolate life of a northern community, where he practiced before his appointment at Baths. Here he has great plans to develop the town into a more fashionable spa center.

As the play opens Dr. Stockman receives a letter from the university to which he had mailed a sample of the city's water. The reply confirms his worst suspicions, which were generated by a rash of stomach ailments and typhoid cases among the previous season's vacationers. But the report is even worse than he had imagined. The town is a cesspool, dangerous to health because of the refuse from the local tanneries, owned, ironically, by his father-in-law. The polluted runoff has affected the water in the pipes that feed the pump room and has seeped out onto the beach where the baths are. He congratulates himself on realizing this in time to prevent more illness, and in turn he is congratulated by his family and friends – one of them a young liberal journalist courting his daughter, Petra. The only solution is to relay the entire water system.

The doctor cannot imagine he will be thwarted in his recommendation, though he is warned by his brother that a project of such magnitude will be very costly and will take two full years to complete, jeopardizing the profitable tourism trade. When Peter orders him to cancel his plan to publish the university reports about the town's water-contamination problem and further threatens him that disobeying may well harm not only him but also his wife and children, Stockman replies: "Even if my whole world crashes about me, I shall never bow my head."[2]

His resolve is soon to be tested as his friends begin to vacillate and the liberal but corrupt journalists withdraw their support. His opportunity to explain his convictions comes at a gathering of citizens at the home of his friend, Captain Hovsted. At first the crowd is sympathetic as he explains that his only ambition is to work for the welfare of his community, but soon he lashes out at the stupidity of the authorities, which stand in his way. His rhetoric heats up:

> "I can't stand politicians! I've had all I can take of them. They're like goats on a plantation of young trees. They destroy everything. They block the way for a free man, however much he may twist and turn – and I'd like to see them rooted out and exterminated, like other vermin."[3]

He begins to rave:

> "The most dangerous enemies of truth and freedom are the majority. Yes, the solid, liberal, bloody majority – they are the ones we have to fear. The majority is never right! Never, I tell you! Who forms the majority in any country? The wise or the fools? I think we'd all have to agree that the fools are in a terrifying, overwhelming majority all over the world. But in the name of God it can't be right that the fools should rule the wise! The majority has the power – unfortunately – but the majority is not right! The ones who are right are a few isolated individuals like me! The minority is always right."[4]

Unable to stop himself, he continues:

> "I intend to start a revolution against the lie that truth is the monopoly of the majority! My whole point is that it is the masses, the mob, the damned majority – they are poisoning the sources of our spiritual life and contaminating the ground we walk on."[5]

It becomes impossible to discuss the matter of water contamination in the town. The deeply offended and furious listeners to Dr. Stockman's diatribes accept, with only one dissenting vote (from a drunk), the resolution that Dr. Stockman is an enemy of the people.

Dr. Stockman wants to escape to the New World but Captain Hovsted's ship is sacked because he is sympathetic to the doctor. The play's end does not resolve how Stockman is going to support himself and his family while staying in the town without a job. His family is persecuted, his house is damaged by the stone-casting mob and he is left with only non-paying patients. What's worse, his father-in-law announces that he had invested the inheritance of his daughter and her children in shares of the Baths. By maintaining that the Baths are polluted, Dr. Stockman will ruin his family. We do not find out what will happen but the doctor's final declaration is: "the fact is, you see, that the strongest man in the world is he who stands most alone."[6]

This is probably Ibsen's least satisfactory ending. And Stockman may be Ibsen's least satisfactory hero. We first see him as a champion for clean water and proper waste disposal, an early environmentalist, a potential Sierra Club member, an opponent of corrupt politicians who try to suppress the truth because they fear tourism will decline. But when faced with opposition he espouses perilous views, challenging the will of the majority and proclaiming that only an aristocratic intellectual elite is capable of correct judgment. Is he a dangerous demagogue or a harmless, impulsive man? There is a basic contradiction when he proclaims that, for him, liberty is the first and highest condition of life, while also maintaining that all who disagree with him do not deserve to live. But these ideas probably express Ibsen's convictions at the time he wrote the play.

The role of Dr. Thomas Stockman in *An Enemy of the People*, a favorite of the influential Russian director Stanislavsky, was coveted by the greatest actors. The play has been the darling of revolutionaries in various societies, particularly in Russia, even though the freedom-championing proclamations of Dr. Stockman are muddled and controversial. The play has to be understood in the context of Ibsen's own ideological outlook. Ten years before it was written, he was asserting that liberals are the worst enemies of freedom and that spiritual and intellectual freedom flourish best under absolutism. Eight years later he complained that the opinion of the majority is wrong. "What is the majority? The ignorant mass! The intelligence is always in the minority. How many in the majority do you think are qualified to hold an opinion? Most of them are just sheep dogs."[7]

As one ponders how a sympathetic, idealistic man dedicated to the welfare of the community becomes an enemy of these people, in Dr. Stockman's case it is contempt, intolerance and arrogance that has brought him down.

## REFERENCES

1 Ibsen H (1882). *An Enemy of the People* in *Henrik Ibsen Plays: two (A Doll's House, An Enemy of the People, Hedda Gabler)*. Translated from the Norwegian and introduced by Michael Meyer. London: Methuen Drama; 1980. pp. 108–222.

2 Ibid., p. 161.

3 Ibid. p. 191.

4 Ibid. pp. 192–3.

5 Ibid. p. 194.

6 Ibid. p. 222.

7 Ibid., Introduction, p. 114.

## PART NINE

# Contemporary doctors

# CHAPTER 24

# Dr. Benjamin Rubin

## in *Open Heart*
### by A.B. Yehoshua[1]

---

### Themes

- Medical mistakes, one from lack of knowledge, the other caused by politics
- Seeking spirituality in India
- Hospital resident contemplates choice of medical specialty
- Young doctor obsessively pursuing an older woman

---

Abraham B. Yehoshua was born in Jerusalem in 1936 in the fifth generation of a Sephardic Jewish family. He is so deeply Israeli that he says, "Diaspora Jews change their nationalities like jackets . . . I cannot keep my identity outside Israel. Being Israeli is in my skin, not on my jacket."[2] Educated at the Hebrew University in literature and philosophy, he taught briefly in Paris in the 1960s and, since 1972, has taught at the University of Haifa, where he is currently a senior lecturer in literature. Probably the best-known Israeli writer outside the country, he has been deeply influenced by Franz Kafka, S.Y. Agnon and William Faulkner. He is a member of the new generation of Israeli writers who moved from the social concerns of earlier authors to focus on the individual and interpersonal, and his fiction has won several Israeli prizes and the 2006 Los Angeles Book Prize for *A Woman in Jerusalem*. Previous widely read novels include *The Lover*, *A Late Divorce*, *Mr. Mani* and *The Liberated Bride*.

## THE NOVEL

We first meet Dr. Benjamin Rubin as he is jockeying for a surgical residency at his hospital in Tel Aviv. Immediately we understand that he's obsessed with becoming a surgeon, and just as quickly we know that his desire will be thwarted because Dr. Hishin, head of the surgery department, obviously prefers the other resident for the one place open for next year. But Hishin, who is familiar with Rubin's laudable performance during his rotation on the internal medicine service, recommends him to the hospital's administrator, Mr. Lazar, to accompany him to India, where Lazar's daughter, Einat, has become ill with acute hepatitis B and needs to be brought home from Gaya, a mid-size town near Varanasi (Benares), which is about 300 miles west of Calcutta. Benjy is at first reluctant to accept this sudden assignment since it will mean missing half of his final month on surgery, but Dr. Hishin advises him to take it – to get to know Lazar if nothing else, since Lazar is influential in medical circles and can help him in the future. Benjy vacillates but finally decides to go, seeing the trip as a chance to take a break from his intensive year without a day off and figure out what to do next with his career.

The plane trip takes him, Lazar and Lazar's wife, Dori, an attractive lawyer in her mid-forties, via Rome to New Delhi, from which they must take a 17-hour train ride to Varanasi, a religious center now overflowing with pilgrims. The spiritual atmosphere fascinates Benjamin. He goes off at once to the river, led by the resilient porter, who puts him in a little boat with two Scandinavian backpackers so that they can watch the rites – funerary, religious, hygienic – from the water. There are women in saris dipping their hair into the water and half-naked men who dive in and emerge purified; pilgrims performing their religious rites while in the background loudspeakers chant long prayers; bathers emerging from the water to do their yoga exercises; and a big red funeral pyre. Benjy approaches the ghat containing the pyre and stares in fascination as the corpse burns. He waits till the fire is out, watching the relatives gathered around the ashes until one of them cracks the skull to liberate the soul and then sprinkles the ashes on the water of the holy river. Somehow he is strangely moved by all this – the spirit of India seems to be taking over. As he tells the skeptical Lazars of his experience he chides them for not coming to the river, just watching from the balcony.

> ". . . there's something very strong here. It's hard to explain. Something very ancient – not like historical ruins in Israel, it's not historical, it's real. If you go down, you'll feel that what's happening here, the purification rites and the cremations, have been going on for thousands of years as if that's the way it's been forever."[3]

On the brief train ride to Gaya they meet two brothers, one a doctor, who tell the Lazars they've heard that the hospital in Gaya is small and poorly equipped and that they should take their daughter at once to Calcutta, where medical care is more reliable, giving them their cards in case they need help. At the hospital they learn that Einat has been moved to Bodhgaya, 10 miles away, a religious retreat full of Buddhist monasteries. They find her lying exhausted in the fetal position on a sleeping bag covered with a gray sheet, attended by two Japanese girls. Rubin observes that her face is pure and fine, her blonde hair cropped, her eyes those of her frail grandmother he had met so briefly, her skin dry and green as bark, her hands restlessly scratching herself because of the itch that is typical of hepatitis. He realizes her condition is not good and that he must perform a blood count and sedimentation rate immediately, check her exact bilirubin and glucose levels, assess her liver function and examine her urine. While Lazar and his wife search for suitable accommodations, Rubin does a physical and finds her heartbeat regular but is barely able to palpate her liver, which seems to have shrunk. Telling himself that it couldn't have begun to degenerate only two months into the disease, he finds her gall bladder enlarged and so tender that she screams when he touches it.

After moving Einat to a local hotel Rubin is apprehensive, fearing an internal hemorrhage because of his inability to palpate her liver. He decides to take the urine and blood samples immediately to Gaya and check out the hospital's equipment, for he remembers the warning of the doctor they met on the train. If the results of the tests are bad, they should move her at once to the Calcutta hospital recommended by the Indian doctor. He leaves cortisone ointment for the itch and paracetamol to bring down the fever. At the Gaya hospital he is assailed by a smell of rot so dank and violent he covers his nose with a gauze pad sprinkled with iodine. He leaves the samples with a tall thin Indian woman who refuses to process them at once – everyone here is sick, she says, everyone wants answers. While waiting for the test results Rubin sees a plane landing and discovers that it stopped on its way to Calcutta. Immediately he decides to take the samples there since he has duplicates of everything and talks his way onto the crowded plane, where they give him a little folding chair to sit on in the back. He must get the results of liver function tests, the two transaminases, the clotting factors, the glucose level. Rubin's suspicions turn out to be right – there is liver damage, the coagulation system is impaired, the bilirubin level very high. Low blood sugar may explain the extreme fatigue. Einat needs an urgent injection of glucose and something to replenish the clotting factors, a blood transfusion. With no time to waste, the doctor and his brother bring Benjy to the night train, which will take him back to his patient by morning.

On his return he immediately gives Einat a shot of glucose, which has a wonderful effect; suddenly she is able to get up and sit with them in the kitchen for a midnight snack. But 12 hours later her condition has again deteriorated. Another shot of glucose helps, but on a walk taken to prepare her for the trip home the next day, she has a nosebleed, suggesting a threat of a more serious hemorrhage. Rubin ascertains that Dori has a compatible blood type in case of need. Another nose bleed on the short flight to Varanasi, plus blood in vomit she throws up at the airport, convince Dr. Rubin he has to stop this trip and arrange for a transfusion with the mother's blood. This he accomplishes meticulously in a room at the Ganges Hotel in Varanasi and, after a 30-hour wait to give Einat time to sleep, they continue to New Delhi. Watching his patient, Rubin is convinced that the transfusion has been vital, as the nosebleeds have stopped completely. But Einat is still febrile and itching.

The first hint questioning Rubin's medical judgment comes after he returns to Israel, and it is from his friend and fellow physician Eyal, who points out he might have infected the mother with the daughter's virus. Rubin says it's impossible; the mother was placed higher than the daughter so there could be no reverse blood flow.

Back at the hospital Hishin tells Rubin that he thinks the transfusion was the correct procedure but that Professor Levine, head of internal medicine and an expert on hepatitis, disagrees. He advises him to see Levine and clear up the transfusion business; then he and Lazar will ask Levine to give him the six-month substitute doctor position that will soon become available in internal medicine. Take it, says Hishin, learn what you can, and if you're still so sure you must be a surgeon, eventually you'll find someone who'll take you back to the operating room. So Dr. Rubin must accept, with that sinking feeling all young physicians experience when the residency of their dreams is not granted, that he may have a different future.

While Rubin is waiting for Levine, who periodically suffers from depression and goes into some unnamed facility to clear his head, Dr. Nakash, the Indian anesthetist who works with Hishin, offers to let Benjy assist him with the anesthesia at operations performed by Hishin at a private hospital.

Rubin finally meets with Dr. Levine, who is adamant that the transfusion wasn't necessary, maintaining that Einat's bleeding stopped on its own, not because of the transfusion, which was completely ineffective because the clotting factors are enzymes not blood cells and behave differently in a transfusion; they're absorbed and disappear unless diluted in a special serum to bind them and prevent this dissolution. This Rubin could not have known without Levine's articles, which Hishin had forgotten to give him in the haste of departure. But what he could have done is infect Dori. Levine advises Rubin to spend the next week in the library learning the elementary laws of physics and reading about how viruses, particularly those causing hepatitis B and C, move and multiply in the bloodstream so that he'll understand how he could have infected a healthy woman for "the sake of your pointless theatrics."[4]

Humiliated, Rubin seeks out Nakash, who soothes him and says, don't worry, Levine is an unhappy man who likes to make others miserable and, anyway, you'll be an anesthesiologist. Subsequently, Lazar offers Benjy a job in England, at St. Bernadine's Hospital, which has a functioning exchange program with their hospital. An English doctor is working in Professor Levine's department, but the Israeli doctor who was supposed to go to London could not get a work permit and Lazar, remembering Benjy's British passport, decides that this 10-month experience will be just right for him.

In England Sir Geoffrey, the administrator at St. Bernadine's, knows of Rubin's surgical desires from Lazar. While the Department of Surgery has no room for him, the ER does. His first operation is on a young girl injured in a car accident; the senior surgeon leaves for another case and Rubin is on his own for the first time in his life. He slowly, very slowly, repairs tears in internal vessels, thinking that perhaps Hishin and Nakash are right about his abilities. But the British doctors have every confidence because of his surgical and military experience and he gets to do a lot of surgery.

The author portrays the medical scenes accurately and with great detail, a remarkable example of which is the coronary artery bypass performed on Mr. Lazar. Unfortunately, for medical-political reasons, the operation is carried out by a more famous scientist but one with less practical experience and a less skillful assisting team. Rubin gets Nakash to let him assist with anesthesia. They use a fentanyl drip rather than anesthetic gases for precise control, and the expert Nakash is so nervous that he mishandles the endotracheal tube insertion and has to correct his error while the cardiac anesthetist calmly inserts an extra intravenous line into Lazar's leg in case of an urgent need for blood or fluids and a long, thin catheter into the penis. Nakash, recovered, inserts the central venous line through the jugular vein into the right atrium of the heart. There is some tension, as the usual routine of assistants doing the initial surgical tasks until the exact moment when the master surgeon sweeps in to work his magic is different here, with Professor Adler actually involved from the start. He opens the chest with Hishin as his assistant, detaches the internal mammary artery and clamps its lower end, immerses the saphenous vein destined to become another conduit in its softening solution, clamps the aortic outlet from the heart, attaches two suction tubes to the inferior vena cava and then connects the tubes of the cardiopulmonary bypass machine, uttering the words "Bypass on" to warn the two technicians to be ready to drive the entire blood circulation through the wheels of the machine so that he can work on the unmoving heart, inserting the venous and arterial bypasses.

The post-operative course is stormy, with ventricular tachycardia degenerating into lethal ventricular fibrillation. The autopsy shows a recent myocardial infarction attributed to a clot in the bypassed coronary artery.

It is difficult to predict what will happen to Dr. Benjamin Rubin. He is a capable physician, well trained in internal medicine, with good surgical hands and experience with anesthesia – seemingly a promise of a successful career of his choice, but we have witnessed the impulsive blood transfusion, which he did without consulting by phone a more experienced specialist. His private life poses more questions about his character. First, during the trip to India he falls in love with Dori Lazar, who is only nine years younger than his mother. This grows into an obsession, perhaps a substitution for his obsession with surgery. His maneuvering brings them together in her mother's apartment and they make passionate love. After she comments that he is too dangerous for her – a bachelor with nothing to lose – he impulsively marries young Michaela, Einat's friend who first brought the news of her illness to the Lazars. She is immersed in Buddhism and just back from India. Michaela, a flower child with a shaven head, becomes pregnant and, when she goes into labor and the midwife fails to appear, Rubin must deliver his own daughter, whom Michaela names Shiva. After Lazar's death, Benjy is convinced that Lazar's soul has entered his body. The transmigration of souls does not surprise Michaela, who warns him that he may lose his own soul. "But I've already lost it, Michaela," says Benjy. For Michaela this is all wonder.

> For before her very eyes an ethereal idea from the India she so adored and longed for was being incarnated, not by a Hindu but by a rational, practical, Western doctor, a moderate man trapped in the mystical seam between body and soul.[5]

After the precious Indian six-armed statue that Einat had given Michaela is accidentally broken, Michaela decides she must return to India to get another. She is serious and immediately makes arrangement for her trip, deciding to take Shiva with her. She invites Benjy to go with her and he thinks perhaps he should: "Maybe in the place where the gorgeous silk of my infatuation had gradually been woven, my love might slowly unravel and dissolve into the mystery that had given birth to it."[6]

But Michaela is unable to use his doubts to sweep him along and he decides he must stay and see this strange compelling love through to whatever end awaits him. The conclusion comes quickly; Dori breaks off the affair, saying she wants to be alone. Soon Benjamin learns from Hishin that she's planning to go to Europe. Meanwhile his parents and he learn that all is not well with Shiva, who has diarrhea that won't clear up. When Benjamin refuses to become alarmed and do anything, his mother takes off without telling him or his father and goes to Calcutta to bring the baby home. In the end we are left wondering whether Benjamin will overcome his strange, obsessive and impossible love and be able to live with Michaela again, and if Michaela, who is now working with the sidewalk doctors in Calcutta, will be able to leave India. As in real life, we don't know what's going to happen next.

In this and several other novels of Yehoshua, sexual obsession plays a large role in the plot, but medicine is a new theme. Here he delivers the profession of medicine two unkindly cuts – a doctor failing to curb his sexual drive and the unnecessary death of a middle-aged man after a routine, ordinarily low-risk procedure – the victim of medical politics. It is wonderfully written with a magic pen but not with an open heart.

## REFERENCES

1 Yehoshua AB (1994). *Open Heart*. New York: Doubleday and Company; 1999.
2 Wikipedia. *A. B. Yehoshua*. Available at: http://en.wikipedia.org/wiki/A._B._Yehoshua. From a speech delivered at the opening panel of the centennial celebration of the American Jewish Committee. *Jerusalem Post*, May 11, 2006.
3 Yehoshua, op. cit., p. 70.
4 Ibid., p. 203.
5 Ibid., p. 420.
6 Ibid., p. 433.

# CHAPTER 25

# Dr. Henry Perowne

## in *Saturday*

### by Ian McEwan[1]

---

### Themes

- What can happen to a fashionable London neurosurgeon in one day
- Rare medical diagnosis made from observing the subject on the street

---

The British novelist Ian McEwan, born in Aldershot in England in 1948, was educated at Eton, the University of Sussex and the University of East Anglia, where he took a creative writing course taught by the novelists Malcolm Bradbury and Angus Wilson.

His first published work was a collection of short stories, *First Love, Last Rites*, which won the Somerset Maugham award in 1976. This was followed by three novels that received some success in the 1980s and early 1990s. The first of his later novels, regarded as masterpieces, was *Enduring Love*, about a person with the rare neurological de Clerambault's syndrome. In 1998 he was awarded the Booker Prize for the novel *Amsterdam*. His book *Atonement* was named by *Time Magazine* the best novel of 2002. The novel *Saturday*, considered by some critics as his best, received the James Tall Black Memorial Prize for 2005.

McEwan has won a reputation as one of Britain's greatest literary minds. He is praised for a concise, thoughtful, elegant and restrained style, though some critics believe that his novels are too structured. His latest book is a slim volume entitled *On Chesil Beach*.

## SATURDAY

The novel records events taking place on a single day, February 15, 2003, in the life of a 48-year-old neurosurgeon, Henry Perowne, who is a senior physician in a teaching hospital in London. His somewhat younger wife, Rosalind, is an attractive lawyer and a writer, the latter talent inherited from her father, the famous poet John Grammaticus, who, after his wife's death, settled in a castle in Southern France. No less talented are the two children of Rosalind and Henry, 21-year-old Daisy, who has just published a book of poems, and 18-year-old Theo, a promising guitarist playing in a touring band. A family reunion of these five people is planned for the evening in the spacious and elegant apartment of the Perownes. Henry is a happily married man; he loves his wife and is proud of the children and his own physical prowess, allowing him to play a brisk game of squash and run a half-marathon each year. The only regret he has is that medicine leaves him no time to read literary works suggested by Daisy. On this particular non-working Saturday his routine includes a squash game with his anesthetist friend, Jay Weiss, a visit to his mother, who is losing the last vestiges of her memory in a home for old people, purchasing ingredients for an elaborate fish stew he will cook tonight, attending the rehearsal of his son's concert, and making love to his wife twice, in the early morning and the late evening. But the day also includes two extraordinary events.

As he awakens at 3:40 a.m. and peers through the window of the living room he sees an airplane with one wing aflame streaking toward Heathrow airport. Later, when he watches the news on TV, he learns that this was a Russian cargo plane on the way from Riga to Birmingham, and that it landed safely, but the image of the handcuffed pilot and co-pilot on the next newscast hints at a possible terrorist action. More important to him personally is a minor car collision, which occurs while driving in his luxurious 500 Mercedes to the squash game. En route he encounters a large protest demonstration against the imminent invasion of Iraq, which forces a diversion of traffic. A busy policeman, overwhelmed by the chaos, allows Henry to turn into a one-way street going in the wrong direction, and his car brushes against an oncoming BMW vehicle. The Mercedes suffers minor scratches on the right side, and the sideboard mirror of the BMW is knocked off. The driver of the BMW with the detached mirror, a pugnacious thug named Baxter, and his two accompanying hoodlums, Nark and Nigel, approach Dr. Perowne and ask for cash to fix the damage. When he refuses on the grounds that it needs to be settled by the insurance companies, the response is a severe blow to his chest which nearly knocks him off his feet. He escapes further thrashing in a curious way. Observing Baxter's twitching face and the coarse tremor of his hands, he suspects that Baxter is afflicted by the hereditary Huntington's chorea, which is lethal in mid-life. Curious about the correctness of his diagnosis, he asks Baxter about his father. The perplexed Baxter is even more baffled by finding out that this man in the rumpled sweatsuit is a doctor, and he lets Henry drive off to his game, but he remains offended, resenting the perceived indignity imposed by the wealthy doctor who penetrated the secrets of his illness.

Baxter reappears in the evening and walks over to Rosalind, who has just returned home, and points a knife at her neck. She receives a little cut to remind the assembled family that Baxter is serious. More damage is done to the nose of John Grammaticus for taunting him. Baxter is accompanied by his pal Nigel. Both behave badly. They demand the surrender of all phones and order drinks. Baxter forces Daisy to undress, which reveals that she is pregnant. He spots the book of her poems and asks her to recite some of them, which somehow changes his mood. He allows Daisy to get dressed and pockets the book. He becomes intrigued when Henry speaks of new therapy for his disease and accompanies him upstairs to retrieve the literature about this new procedure. This provides an opportunity for Henry and Theo to jump on Baxter, disarm him and push him down the stairway. Baxter's head hits the floor; he suffers a concussion and skull fracture and is transported by an arriving ambulance to Henry's hospital emergency room. Later Dr. Perowne receives a call from his anesthetist friend asking him to operate on Baxter because the complexity of the traumatic injury requires unusually skillful handling.

> Perowne takes a look at Baxter's head to make sure Rodney [the registrar] shaved him in exactly the right place. The laceration is straight and clean – a wall, a skirting board, a stone-floor landing rather than the grit and filth you see in wounds after road traffic accidents – and has been sown up by A and E. Even without touching, he can see the top of his patient's head has an area of boggy swelling – blood is collecting between the bone and the scalp.[2]

This and other details of this operation and the diagnosis of Huntington's chorea made on the street are but a few displays of the author's diligently acquired knowledge of neurology and neurosurgery. From his days as a registrar Henry recounts a case of the surgical removal of a hypophyseal tumor pressing on the optic chiasm and nearly blinding a young law student, who becomes his wife and the only love of his life. Further recollections involve other procedures, such as clipping the neck of a middle cerebral artery aneurysm, craniotomy for a meningioma and resection of a pilocytic astrocytoma. This approach of showing off the author's knowledge of human anatomy, pathology, biochemistry and genetics can be appreciated by the medical profession but is way above the heads of lay readers. It is not surprising, therefore, that it was ignored in all published reviews available to us, and that the reviewers tended to concentrate on family interactions and on the way we live today.

Subjecting this enjoyable reading to a stricter scrutiny, we recognize a skillfully constructed collage from newspaper clippings, TV images and excerpts from medical textbooks. We are reminded that a single error of judgment can have devastating consequences. But this is nothing new. Similarly there is no surprise in Daisy's accurate forecasting of what will happen in Iraq after the invasion.

Comparing this day with James Joyce's June 16, 1904, when Bloom roamed the streets of Dublin, or with Solzhenitsyn's *One Day in the Life of Ivan Denisovich*, revealing the horrors of Soviet gulag, would be an unpardonable sacrilege.

**REFERENCES**

1 McEwan I. *Saturday*. New York: Anchor Books; 2005.
2 Ibid., p. 257. No permission required by the publisher.

# Reprint permissions for copyrighted material

# Index